D0867304

the {*strangest*} song

the {*strangest*} song

One Father's Quest
to Help His Daughter Find Her Voice

Teri Sforza
with Howard and Sylvia Lenhoff

*The Compelling Story of the Link between a
Rare Genetic Disorder and Musical Talent*

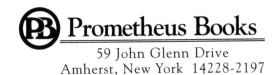

Prometheus Books

59 John Glenn Drive
Amherst, New York 14228-2197

Inquiries should be addressed to
Prometheus Books
59 John Glenn Drive
Amherst, New York 14228–2197
VOICE: 716–691–0133, ext. 207
FAX: 716–564–2711
WWW.PROMETHEUSBOOKS.COM

10 09 08 07 06   5 4 3 2 1

Library of Congress Cataloging-in-Publication Data

Sforza, Teri.
    The strangest song : one father's quest to help his daughter find her voice / by Teri
Sforza, with Howard and Sylvia Lenhoff.
        p. cm.
    Includes bibliographical references and index.
    ISBN 13: 978-1-59102-478-1 (hardcover : alk. paper)
    ISBN 10: 1-59102-478-1 (hardcover : alk. paper)
    1. Lenhoff, Gloria—Health. 2. Williams syndrome—Patients—Biography. I.
Lenhoff, Howard. II. Lenhoff, Sylvia. III. Title.
    RJ506.W44.S46 2006
    362.198'9200092—dc22

[B]2006020198

Printed in the United States on acid-free paper

Every attempt has been made to trace accurate ownership of copyrighted material
in this book. Errors and omissions will be corrected in subsequent editions,
provided that notification is sent to the publisher.

We dedicate this book to the teachers, musicians, and maestros who recognize the musical abilities of the intellectually disabled, and find ways to help them shine; to the parents who make exceptional efforts so their musically abled, intellectually disabled children get advanced musical training; and to the talented, gutsy musicians who are devoting years to study and practice. Their performances bring pleasure to all who hear them, and hope to families of disabled children.

{*contents*}

{acknowledgments}

Deep and profound thanks to Gloria, John, Alec, Brian, Meghan, Ben, Chris, Charles, and all the other absolutely amazing Williams syndrome people I've had the honor and pleasure of meeting over the years of researching this book. They are truly an inspiration and a wonder, and remind us all of the power inherent in every human being. Extra special thanks to Sharon Libera for her vision, fabulous memory, sharp editing pen, and amazing record keeping; Kay Bernon, Terry Monkaba, Lori Sweazy, Liz and Bob Costello, Bob Ackley, Nancy Goldberg, and all the other parents and activists for sharing their triumphs and struggles; the scientists who generously gave their time to make sure I correctly interpreted their work, including Dan Levitin, Audrey Don, Colleen Morris, Paul Wang, Helen Tager-Flusberg, Ursula Bellugi, Annette Karmiloff-Smith, Melissa Rowe, Olegario Perales, and Gregory Hickok; Arlene Alda, James Maas, Greg Detweiler, Dalit Warshaw, and all the other keen observers who shared their fascination with the syndrome; UCLA professors Richard Walter, Hal Ackerman, Howard Suber, and Lew Hunter for drilling story structure into my head; Betsy Amster, for believing in the story; Rebecca Allen, for her thoughtful edit; Joan and Murray Light, my editor-and-writer in-laws, whose book let us cross paths with Paul Kurtz; my husband, Jeff, for not editing me into madness; Jian and Dat Vang, for taking care of our darling daughter, Xia, while I wrote; my late mom, Marie Sforza, for insisting I go to college while my dad was pushing for secretarial school; my dad, Peter, for giving in, and for appreciating Mom in the end; and dear Xia herself. My greatest wish is that she will live up to her full potential, like the amazing people in these pages.

— Teri Sforza

Our daughter, Gloria, and other musically gifted individuals with Williams-Beuren syndrome (WBS) have benefited from the insight, faith, commitment, and varied talents of many supporters. With grateful hearts we salute some of them here and ask the forgiveness of others not mentioned who also have helped.

First we thank Nancy Goldberg, director of the Belvoir Terrace Music Camp in Lenox, Massachusetts. Upon meeting Gloria and Williams musician John Libera in the summer of 1993, Nancy immediately recognized their uncanny talent and took on the highly experimental challenge of sponsoring at Belvoir Terrace a weeklong music camp expressly tailored for the musically able, intellectually impaired campers with Williams-Beuren syndrome. Without Nancy's expertise and involvement, the gifts of our Williams-Beuren syndrome musicians likely would be viewed still as the quaint behavior of a few individuals "compensating for their genetic anomaly."

Our next key figure is Kay Bernon, chairperson of the board of the Berkshire Hills Music Academy (BHMA) in South Hadley, Massachusetts. Kay, a smart, sensitive, and savvy parent of a son, Charles, with WBS, has given years of dedication, using her organizational and fund-raising skills to create the BHMA and have it become the leading institution promoting the development of musical skills and musical vocations for the intellectually impaired.

Were it not for the insight and artistry of Arlene Alda and Professor James Maas, and their production of the award-winning public television documentary *Bravo, Gloria*, our introduction to the world of Williams syndrome might have been delayed for years.

Others were important links in the chain of support leading to the work of Nancy and Kay. Gordon Biescar, as founder and first president of the Williams Syndrome Foundation, gathered a group of parents who, beyond focusing their energies on the difficult problems of raising children with WBS, forged new approaches to deal with research and long-term residences, and eventually the establishment of the Belvoir weeklong camp and the BHMA. Howard, visiting his aging mother, Goldie Lenhoff, in Massachusetts, organized a meeting in Boston of WBS parents interested in advanced music education for their children. Within a day of that meeting he learned of Nancy Goldberg from his high school friend and a business associate of Nancy's, Robert Bashevkin. The events came fast during the following years with much help from such parents and from the Williams Syndrome Association. We thank them all.

We thank Teri Sforza for lending her writing skills and interest in Williams syndrome to make this book possible. We are happy that we could offer our help and comments for the prelude, chapters 1–3, 5–9, 11, 13–15, the coda, and appendices A and B.

For her journey to becoming a professional musician, Gloria needed and had the support, counsel, and friendship of many FOGS, "Friends of Gloria." Special among them were her "Best Buddy," Suzie Motinishi Greenbaum, Nancy Levin, cousin Joe Malatsky, Jessica Stanford, Hillary Kaye, Rosemarie Hallack, Aunt Barbara Schwartz and her family, and the Sklar extended family of Baltimore; the DeLacy, Gobbis, Greeley, Kahn, Karni,

Lasher, Ngo, Rosener, Schwartz, Shishkoff, Sklansky, Somers, Tyler, and Weiland families of Orange County, California; the Carter, Jackson, Kiniery, Munger, Root, Sands, Seward, and Shinn families of Crescent City, California; and the staff of her home at the Baddour Center, Senatobia, Mississippi.

Gloria's maternal grandmother, Dora Grossman, charmed her granddaughter from early childhood with many Hebrew, Yiddish, and old-time songs. Gloria's talented and devoted brother, Bernie, taught her fine points of music and performance and produced her first five cassettes. Creative neighbor Stephen DeLacy designed her DVDs. Ann Wilson of Miami first recognized Gloria's potential as a lyric soprano and how she might learn demanding classical music without needing to read musical notation. In California, junior high music teacher Luella Dick encouraged Gloria's singing, and music therapist Richard Kuykendall declared at her audition that she did not need therapy; she needed vocal instruction. He proceeded to engage her in a broad repertoire of lieder, religious, and operatic music. After he left town, Gloria was ready for the teaching and coaching of university music faculty. In California we are deeply indebted to Barbara Hasty. At the University of Mississippi, Gregory Rike, Herbert V. Jones, Diane Wang, and Sherry Styers broadened Gloria's repertoire and groomed her as a professional classical vocal talent. Our thanks to Oklahoma Professor Sandra Meyers, who accompanied Gloria in concerts and on their *Music-Minus-One* CD.

Honing of accordion skills first came from Marc Moreels and Sigfried Kukier, students at the University of California, Irvine. Dutch American accordionist Roek Willemze brought Gloria professional expertise and a wide and varied approach to the instrument. In Los Angeles, Paul Levoe introduced Gloria to the MIDI and the electronic accordion, and big band accordionist Danny Gould helped broaden Gloria's Broadway and Hollywood repertoire. In Oxford, Mississippi, her accordion performances have gained new southern twists under the tutelage of Ms. Gaye Calhoun.

The door to Jewish liturgy and song was opened for Gloria by her bat mitzvah instructor at Beth David Congregation in Miami, Mr. Louis Gadon. Later, in California, Nora Nissan and Sylvia Haas led her further. From Yochi Levine in Rehovot, Israel, she learned a treasury of Hebrew folk music; at Congregation B'nai Israel in Tustin, California, in the choir under Cantor Hal Hurwitz, Gloria learned more of the High Holiday Hebrew liturgy; and with Cantor David Julian of Memphis, she continues with the delights of the Judaic repertoire. In Tupelo, Mississippi, Temple B'nai Israel leader Marc Perler and Cantor Donald Kartiganer welcome Gloria as assistant cantor. For the songs Gloria sings in thirty languages with near native accents, she is indebted to Steve Berman of Ashland, Oregon, and to a number of her father's fine immigrant students at the University of California. Jill Dovre of Crescent City, California, has helped bring the opera-infatuated Gloria into the realms of pop, rock, and folk. From Jackson, Mississippi, blues star Dorothy Moore and Marcia Weaver of Jackson's "Bach to Blues" have offered encouragement, affection, and performance platforms.

Three "divas" have played roles in Gloria's continuing love affair with opera: Suzanna Guzmann (Los Angeles Opera) and Jacqueline Zander (Boston Lyric Opera) have performed with her, and Sharon Dobbins (Opera Memphis) has become a true mentor. Choral directors James Frieman, Martin Wright, and Bill Jones have welcomed her into their ensembles.

Special thanks to Dr. Joe Young of the National Science Foundation for taking the gamble that biochemist Howard Lenhoff could make the transition to investigating absolute pitch in Williams people, and to Professor Gregory Hickok and Olegario Perales for collaborating in that fascinating study. We are grateful to associate editor Ricki Rusting of *Scientific American* magazine for helping us catapult the story of the link between music and Williams syndrome to a large international audience, and to leading Williams syndrome research colleagues Colleen Morris and Paul Wang for coediting with Howard the first compendium of research papers on Williams-Beuren syndrome, including two on music, and Johns Hopkins medical editor, Wendy Harris, for publishing it.

Finally, we applaud the maestros in Gloria's life. Conductor David Amos had Gloria solo with the Tifereth Israel Community Orchestra (San Diego's community orchestra), and with the San Diego Master Chorale for three seasons. After she moved to northern Mississippi, composer Michael Ching, artistic director of Opera Memphis, saw way past her disabilities and found her capable of singing professionally with his company in major operas. Bravo and thank you, maestros!

—Howard and Sylvia Lenhoff

Note to the Reader: This book draws on myriad source materials, from scientific papers to documentary films to newspaper articles to people's sometimes-differing recollections of events. Quotes that were recounted secondhand do not appear in quotation marks. Quotes that were made directly—either to Sforza, the Lenhoffs, or were published, recorded, or broadcast—appear in quotation marks. The source material for each chapter is listed in the bibliography at the end of this book.

{prelude}

She squints hard into the spotlight's glare. Her eyesight is poor—part of the syndrome—but she senses the audience rising like a wave, somewhere beyond the footlights.

She's sensitive to sound—part of the syndrome, too. But when the applause explodes, she doesn't clap her hands over her ears the way she might if it was thunder. This is different. A standing ovation. At the Kennedy Center. In Washington, DC. She bows deeply, a genuine diva, and it feels, quite simply, like love. A shower of unconditional, adoring love. She drinks in the adulation with such joy that her grin crinkles her puffy eyes, wrinkles her elfin nose, and exposes each tooth in her wide, expansive mouth.

These are marks of the syndrome as well.

Gloria Lenhoff can't make change for a dollar, or subtract five from twelve, or tell left from right. She can't cross the street alone, or write her name legibly, or read music.

But Gloria Lenhoff can sing like few people in the world can sing, with a classically trained lyric soprano and a repertoire of thousands of songs in Italian, French, German, Japanese, Chinese, Macedonian, Korean, Hungarian, Yiddish, and many other languages. Since she can't read music, each note, each word, each nuance, is stored in her brain, which is only 80 percent as large as yours or mine.

"Deh vieni, non tardar, o gioia bella," she sings beneath the hot lights of the Kennedy Center's Millennium Stage, her rich-as-

15

butter vibrato wrapping around the flirty aria from Mozart's *Le Nozze di Figaro* (*The Marriage of Figaro*). "*Vieni ove amore per goder t'appella, Finchè non splende in ciel notturna face, Finchè l'aria è ancor bruna e il mondo tace. . . .*"

She becomes Susanna, taunting Figaro for doubting her fidelity. "Come, do not delay, oh bliss, Come where love calls thee to joy, While night's torch does not shine in the sky, While the air is still dark and the world is quiet. . . ."

This showcase of musicians with disabilities ends with hugs and handshakes, a postperformance reception, toasts in her honor. Ask her how she feels about the music, and she'll tell you in no uncertain terms: "Mozart is fun, but my favorite opera is really *La Bohème* by Giacomo Puccini. I love Puccini."

Gloria Lenhoff has Williams syndrome. Her IQ is fifty-five. She's not supposed to be able to do this.

{chapter 1}

A BABY IS BORN

It was a fine classical guitar, blond and broad-necked, with a tone as rich and smooth and warm as melted chocolate. Howard Lenhoff was not a particularly gifted guitarist, and he knew it. Frankly, he preferred oil painting, which he had dabbled in before. Before Gloria. Before his daughter's birth had obliterated so much of what he recognized from his life. The easel, the brushes, the paints, they would be an impossibility in their claustrophobic apartment, nothing more than quarry for the baby's demolition derby. He yearned for an outlet, an escape, something to soothe his fractured, frazzled nerves; he was only twenty-six, but he was exhausted. The year since Gloria's birth had been the most interminable, agonizing year of his life.

He settled onto the sofa, turning pegs and plucking strings to bring the guitar into tune. A room away, Gloria snapped to attention, as if the sound were a bolt of electricity. She dropped her favorite toy—a jingly key chain she would shake and shake until Howard wanted to scream—and crawled as fast as she could to her father's feet, hauling herself up and standing almost on top of him, her nose practically pressed up against the guitar strings, watching, listening, with almost comical intensity. Howard strummed Elizabethan folk songs, classical pieces, sea yarns, cowboy tunes. Gloria stared wide-eyed at the strings the entire time, hypnotized, mesmerized by their luscious sound.

Gloria was never like other children.

Their odyssey began on February 11, 1955. Howard got the phone call at the lab, where he was working his first job as a research biochemist. He rushed to the hospital's nursery and peered through a pane of glass at the squirming bundle in the bassinet marked with his name. She was as tiny and wrinkled and fragile as a newborn bird, dark hair plastered to her skull like new feathers, deep indents on either side of her head bearing testimony to the difficult delivery and the doctor's decision to wrench her from the birth canal with forceps. His daughter—to spoil, to sing with, to walk down the aisle on her wedding day. Howard stared at the impossibility of her face: so round, so pink, with a pug nose and a tiny mouth that opened wide in an insistent cry. She didn't look like Sylvia, his wife. She didn't look like him. She looked, actually, like a tiny, angry elf. So very small, he could cup her entire body in the palms of his hands. Weighing just 5.5 pounds. It made him worry. But the doctors reassured him: she came fully equipped with ten fingers, ten toes, legs that kicked and arms that waved.

His daughter. Would she be sweet and studious like Sylvia? Or curious and keen like him? Would her eyes be green, like Sylvia's, or nearly black, like his? Would she love science and history and do well in school and make her parents proud, as they had? Would she be healthy? And happy? Howard and Sylvia decided to call her Gloria, in memory of Howard's beloved grandmother Geeta, whose name means "good" in Yiddish. If only she could see this, Howard thought. Geeta had been Howard's best friend in the crowded wood-frame house where he grew up in "the Swamp" of North Adams, Massachusetts. She spoke mainly Yiddish, having fled the pogroms in Latvia, and encouraged her mischievous grandson as he transformed the attic into a laboratory, created homemade fireworks from flash powders, and set off explosions trying to hydrogenate oil to make homemade Crisco. Geeta indulged Howard's obsession with books on chemistry and natural history, and when he became the first member of the Lenhoff family to be accepted into college, she wept with pride. Geeta died two years before Howard earned his bachelor's degree in chemistry, leaving him her most meaningful piece of jewelry: her wedding ring. For years Howard couldn't bring himself to wear it, but on the day he graduated, he slipped it onto his left pinky finger and felt as if she were with him, as if she knew, as if he had made her proud. The ring never left his finger after that day, and he fiddled with it as he gazed at his new baby through the hospital nursery's window. Overwhelmed by the continuity of past, present, and future, he whispered, "Hello, my little Geeta."

Gloria was healthy in all respects, their pediatrician said, except for her small size and a slight heart murmur. Nothing to worry about. Just something to keep an eye on.

The first few weeks a baby comes home are always a jumble of heaven and hell, but this hell had a special fury. Day, night, fed, hungry, Gloria was cranky beyond all imagining, kicking her legs, flailing her arms, and turning bright red as she screamed. It was an insistent cry, a despondent cry, inconsolable and filled with misery. Eating led to violent vomiting, and tiny Gloria lost weight.

Terrible colic, the doctors said. Be patient. She'll outgrow it.

There was only one bedroom in their tiny Connecticut apartment, and the flowered curtains drawn around the bassinet in the corner did nothing to block out the noise. So in the dead of night, one of them paced the floors, bouncing Gloria, trying to quiet the bawling so the other parent could steal enough sleep to function the next day. Howard's work was one of the most important things in the world to him, and sleep deprivation certainly wasn't helping him do his best.

Howard and Sylvia were engaged in 1953, the year that James Watson and Francis Crick announced their discovery of DNA, the chemical code dictating life. Howard was the sort of person who could work himself into fits of passion over biochemistry and its infinite possibilities; he stood on the cutting edge of a revolution that would transform humanity's understanding of the living world, knowledge that would literally unlock the secrets of life, and he knew it. His excitement was infectious as he leaned forward with wide eyes, explaining his research—how tiny traces of metals allow cells to transfer electrons and create the energy that powers existence, how the tiny freshwater hydra might someday help us understand normal and abnormal embryonic development.

Now it was hydra by day, screaming by night. Sometimes, Howard would blast classical music to try to drown it out. Other times, he tied strong twine from Gloria's carriage to his rocking chair, so he could at least sit down and rock her at the same time. When that wasn't enough, he headed to the car and took long drives into the countryside to lull her to sleep. Stopping for red lights and stop signs would only awaken her; so he and Sylvia held their breath and scanned the intersections as their car breezed through.

The walls of the tiny apartment pressed in. Was it only a year ago that they were in Baltimore and Boston, attending plays and concerts? Was it only two years ago that Howard had quoted, from memory, the writings of seventeenth-century scientist and philosopher Blaise Pascal? "Man is but a reed, the most feeble thing in nature, but he is a thinking reed." All our dignity, then, consists in thought. Let us endeavor then, to think well; this is the principle of morality.

Thinking well had seemed so terribly important, but now it

was hard to think at all. Yet they came from steely stock, and they tried to remember that as their eyes burned from lack of sleep. Certainly this was no harder than what their parents and grandparents had endured, fleeing pogroms and poverty in eastern Europe and journeying across the Atlantic in search of a better life in America. No sacrifice was too great for the next generation, their parents had taught them. And there was no greater *nachas*—happiness, reward—than the cry of a child.

How could they complain about one tiny, cranky baby?

Gloria's weight loss continued. The doctors had no idea why. Her features also became more pronounced: Her almond eyes were set in lids so puffy that she looked, from a distance, as exhausted as her parents. Her upturned nose was so pronounced she resembled a little elf. She looked nothing like Sylvia or Howard, or anyone in either family, that anyone could recall.

Gloria kept missing milestones. At two months, most babies can sleep for five or six hours at a stretch. Gloria still awoke, screaming, every two hours. At five months, most babies have doubled their birth weight. Gloria had gained only a couple of pounds. At six months, most babies can sit up by themselves. Gloria was weak, and still had to be propped up. By seven or eight months, most babies are babbling in elaborate invented languages. Gloria made just a few sounds.

Perhaps it was a result of Gloria's early eating difficulties. Now that Gloria was on soy formula and the colic wasn't so bad, maybe Gloria would sleep better, and grow.

Howard never said anything to the contrary. But every time he looked at his daughter, he knew something was wrong. And he felt it was their fault. What mistake had they made? Was it the way the doctor induced labor and broke the amniotic sac, at least one month early? Was it the forceps he used to pull Gloria from the birth canal? The nothing-to-worry-about heart murmur? What could have made their baby turn out this way? What?

The road between their apartment in Stamford and the research lab in Greenwich was wild, green, and winding, studded with small shimmering ponds that reflected the pale winter sky. This drive was one of Howard's few chances to be alone with his emotions and to be brutally honest with himself. He would pull off the road, park the 1953 Plymouth beside one of the ponds, and sob. He was a biologist, damn it. He was supposed to understand. And he understood nothing. He blamed himself and his ignorance of the human embryo for what had happened to Gloria. Somehow he could have, should have, prevented it. Now their baby would suffer, they would suffer, and nothing would ever again be the way it used to be.

Howard retreated into his research, spending more and more time at the lab with his hydras. When he was home, he'd feed Gloria, or rock her, but he couldn't bring himself to help Sylvia with the Sisyphean chores of changing diapers and washing them by hand. It made him nauseated.

Gloria did not take her first steps at age one, as most babies do, and was still sleeping only two or three hours at a stretch. But something delightful was beginning to emerge in her that made the burden easier to bear: she loved to be cuddled and was forever crawling into Howard's or Sylvia's lap, anxious for a reading of *The Cat in the Hat* or *Mother Goose Rhymes*. She could listen to *The Owl and the Pussycat* and "Ba Ba Black Sheep" over and over again—rhythm and rhyme delighted her. She was spellbound by anything that spun—records, tops, clothes in a dryer—and would watch them, frozen with fascination. She was also turning into a charming socialite: when the Lenhoffs had visitors—which was more and more often now—Gloria would crawl fearlessly into the strangers' laps and study the minutiae of their faces, as if the eyebrows and the lips and the chin were the most fascinating and unusual things that ever existed. In the grocery store, Gloria shouted greetings and threw her little arms out to hug the cashier and strangers in the checkout line. Her hair was growing into moppy curls, her smile was punctuated with adorable dimples, and she giggled with delight whenever people paid her any attention. She was, in short, becoming irresistible.

She was also starting to show an acute sensitivity to sound. When Howard and Sylvia played their records—classical and blues LPs, mail ordered from Macy's and Sam Goody for a dollar each—Gloria grew excited and focused all at once, pulling herself up in her crib, holding onto the railings, and bouncing up and down on her stiff little feet, keeping time to the beat. She grimaced when she heard particularly loud cracks of thunder, exploding firecrackers, or screaming police sirens; when balloons burst, she wailed. They worked with this sensitivity, buying her toys that made pretty noises—bells, rattles, little xylophones— and began to realize they could use it to help Gloria learn. With Gloria on the floor at one end of the living room, Sylvia would sit on the floor at the other end, jingle-jangling her keys. The bright metallic ringing proved irresistible to Gloria, who finally perched on her tippy-toes and propelled herself forward to get at them. Success! It was an odd walk, an awkward walk, as Gloria bounced on the balls of her feet and never used her heels; but it was a walk nonetheless. At eighteen months old, Gloria had finally taken her first steps.

They were visiting family in Baltimore when it came time for Gloria's regular checkup. Sylvia made an appointment with the longtime family physician, the one who had attended to Sylvia's own colds and cuts as a child. She watched as the doctor listened to Gloria's heart, peered into her ears and eyes, manipulated her stiff little limbs. In addition to the heart murmur and funny gait, it turned out that Gloria had a partially "frozen" joint in the elbow of her right arm. The doctor measured her, weighed her, considered her quietly. Finally, he said: "She'll never go to Goucher."

Goucher College was Sylvia's alma mater, before she pursued graduate studies at Harvard. The doctor didn't know exactly what was wrong with Gloria. But something was clearly wrong. Sylvia quickly thanked him, bundled Gloria up, and never went back to him again.

The problem was, no one knew exactly what was wrong with Gloria. There was a long list of symptoms—heart murmur, frozen elbow, failure to grow and thrive, delays walking and talking—but never a definitive cause. Howard and Sylvia wanted more children, but they worried. What if it was genetic? What if they had another handicapped baby? Could they live with themselves? Was it selfish to want to try? They confessed their fears to Gloria's regular pediatrician, and he comforted them with statistics: The chances of having two handicapped children in the same family are exceedingly slim, he said. It might actually help Gloria to have a little brother or sister who was developing at a regular pace, and it would do Howard and Sylvia a world of good. He urged them to have another child soon.

The family moved to Washington, DC, in the summer of 1956. Howard, now an officer in the air force, became chief of the biochemistry section of the new Armed Forces Institute of Pathology. There, he delved deeper into his studies on the tentacle-headed hydra, a microscopic organism with a fascinating ability to repair injuries by regeneration. Slice a hydra's body into pieces, and each piece will grow into a new, complete hydra. How did they do that? And what could Howard learn about their behavior and biochemistry that might be applied to understanding humans?

The Institute of Pathology was on the Walter Reed Army Hospital base, and one of the perks was access to some of the best doctors in the nation's capital. A team of thirteen physicians examined Gloria and tried to determine, once and for all, what was wrong. A dizzying number of tests stretched over four days—karyotype chromosomal analysis, blood tests examining major ions and proteins, motor tests, body measurements, psychological tests, x-rays. After nearly a week of conferences and cross-checking, the doctors reached a sobering conclusion: Gloria had suffered brain damage due to a temporary lack of oxygen during the birth process. Take her home and love her, they said. There's nothing you can do differently now.

Brain damage. Lack of oxygen. During birth.

Friends tried to console them. "At least you didn't have a boy," one said, as if having a disabled daughter was somehow more merciful than having a disabled son. Howard choked on bitterness for doctors in general and for the doctor who delivered Gloria in particular; but Sylvia was pregnant again, and her deepest concern at the moment was for the baby she carried. So far, it seemed incomprehensibly easy: no nausea, no bleeding gums, no edema, none of the suffering she endured carrying Gloria. Statistically speaking, this should be a perfectly healthy baby. But was it?

Bernie was born as Gloria's second birthday approached. His eyes were not puffy. His nose was not upturned. He was a solid seven pounds, not tiny and frail as a bird. He did not cry and wiggle and fuss, and he suckled easily and demandingly, so unlike his sister. Clearly, he was a regular, normal, healthy baby.

At home, Bernie became a celebrity. Gloria was fascinated with him and would hover, inches from his face, examining his eyes, his nose, his mouth, his ears, his chin, as if she were trying to memorize every last inch of him. Bernie could not have been a more different baby from Gloria: He did not scream. He slept soundly from the moment he got home, even though his crib was in a busy hallway in the small apartment. He ate well, put on weight, giggled, thrived. Where Gloria hit all the developmental milestones late, Bernie hit them early, quickly closing the distance between himself and his big sister until it seemed, sometimes, that he was the older child. Sylvia would put them on the living room floor and give them their run of toys: puppets, rattles, music boxes, plastic telephones, and Bernie would instruct Gloria on how to play the games he spontaneously invented. After dinner, the dining room table transformed into a stage, where Gloria and Bernie hammed it up with impromptu shows of song and dance for their applauding parents.

Gloria didn't get the toys most kids got. There were no chess or checker games for her, as the rules were too complex; the intricacies of Monopoly, Scrabble, and Parcheesi were far beyond her. Her difficulties with balance and muscle development left many childhood staples out of the question. Almost by default, Gloria's toys became musical. Tambourines, flutophones, drums, xylophones, toy pianos—Sylvia and Howard made sure she got one for every birthday, and they welcomed the resulting din as Gloria banged and blew with abandon. The noise might have driven others to distraction, but it was deeply satisfying for them; here was something their daughter, who usually couldn't concentrate for more than a few minutes at a time, could do for hours. It was obvious that music made Gloria happier than anything else; when she listened as Howard played the guitar or Sylvia played the piano, her face was very close to radiant. That look never crossed her face at any other time.

Bernie raced ahead of Gloria in things like reading and math. While Gloria knew the whole alphabet song by heart, Bernie understood that the letters represented sounds and figured out how to string them together to make words. He was reading cereal boxes and street signs before kindergarten, years before his sister could do the same. Bernie could count how many blocks he had and tell you how many there would be if two were added or taken away, but Gloria couldn't grasp the concept of numbers, no matter how hard Howard and Sylvia tried to make her understand. Bernie understood concepts like "same" and "different," "more" and "less," "big" and "bigger," while Gloria couldn't fathom one from the other, her attention inevitably wandering to the window, to the people, to the voices she heard beyond the apartment walls. Bernie could hold a pencil and draw a passable circle when he was three; a square when he was four; and a triangle when he was five; as well as pictures of people, houses, flowers, and dogs, and raw but recognizable attempts at letters and numbers. Gloria could do none of it. She didn't have the motor control to hold a pencil properly. Her scribbles were indecipherable.

Whatever joy Howard and Sylvia took in Bernie's successes was more than tempered by Gloria's struggles. This is how it would be.

♪ ♪ ♪

The fledgling Howard Hughes Medical Institute was flourishing in Miami in 1958. It was an entirely new and incredibly eclectic endeavor, much like its founder, who did everything from dabble in movies to design, construct, and race airplanes. Hughes would make TWA a major international airline and build the Hughes Aircraft Company into one of America's largest defense contractors. In 1953—the year Watson and Crick discovered DNA— Hughes founded a medical institute largely as a tax shelter and gave it an extraordinary mission: probe the genesis of life itself.

Howard's work on the simple hydra had come to the institute's attention. At the Armed Forces Institute of Pathology, Howard made an important discovery: hydra contain a form of collagen— the fibrous protein essential to forming connective tissues like tendon, sinew, and bone—that had never been identified before. The discovery impressed an expert at the Massachusetts Institute of Technology, and when that expert heard that Hughes was looking for a collagen biochemist for its research cardiology program, he recommended Howard. Howard won a plum assignment as a Howard Hughes investigator, and the family moved to Coral Gables, Florida, a grand Mediterranean Revival city built on what used to be citrus groves on the outskirts of Miami. It was a vibrant place filled with vibrant people, and Gloria quickly set out to meet her new neighbors. She would toddle down the block on the balls of her feet, introducing herself to strangers, asking questions, doling out hugs generously and indiscriminately. Gloria befriended Leni, the Bavarian woman next door, and was soon singing songs in German (*"Hoppe, hoppe Reiter, Wen sie felt dann schre-it'se..."*). She attempted knitting with Ade Brito, the Cuban refugee who worked in The Knit Shop in the tony downtown, and was soon exchanging pleasantries in Spanish (*"Buenas tardes, amigo! Cómo está?"*). She haunted the house down the street, where the family was from Greece, and was soon reciting poems in Greek (*"Apó poú eísaste?"*). And when Sylvia's mother came to live with them, Gloria greedily picked up bits of Yiddish (*"Eli, Eli, lama azavtani?"*), Polish (*"Jak sie masz?"*) and even Italian (*"Buon-giorno! Come stai?"*). Gloria was ravenous for language, any language, collecting words the way other children collect dolls and balls. The spongelike way she absorbed them perplexed Howard and Sylvia; how could she grasp pieces of all these languages while still not grasping simple concepts like "early" and "late"?

After Sylvia took a part-time job teaching at the University of Miami, she enrolled Gloria and Bernie in nursery school at the Young Men's Hebrew Association. When Sylvia dropped them off, Bernie grew quiet, leery of being left with strangers; but Gloria smiled delightedly, waved bye-bye, and set off to meet new people. Sometimes, Sylvia would stand at the gate and watch them. Gloria gravitated to the adults, not to the children. While Bernie and the rest of the children assembled for a circle game, Gloria would wander away to explore the sandbox or the swings. When Bernie and the rest of the children were playing ball games, Gloria would wander away to meet the mailman or sit on a teacher's lap. She didn't like the balloons that appeared on birthdays because their popping unnerved her; she didn't like firecrackers or fireworks on the Fourth of July; she didn't like radios to be turned up too loud. She couldn't stay still, couldn't concentrate, couldn't be like the other children. She just didn't fit in. Sylvia knew they had to do something with Gloria, for Gloria. But she had no idea what.

As Gloria's sixth birthday approached, an eccentric doctor halfway around the world was playing his own game of connect the dots.

Dr. J. C. P. Williams was the registrar at Greenlane Hospital in Auckland, New Zealand, in 1961. He had several children coming in for heart surgery and noticed that they shared a strange, similar narrowing of the aorta, the main artery leading from the heart. It prevented the heart valve from opening and closing properly, obstructing blood flow and causing terrible problems.

The similarities didn't stop there. The children Dr. Williams was seeing looked strangely alike, even though they weren't related. They were small and fine-boned with striking facial features—upturned noses, sharp chins, and haunting eyes that often had white, lacy, snowflake patterns in the iris. They were chatty and outgoing but had mental handicaps, sometimes profound ones. Williams followed up with the hospital's cardiac consultants and was given the go-ahead to investigate further. He wrote an article with the tongue-tying title "Supravalvular aortic stenosis," which appeared in the medical journal *Circulation* that year, describing the perplexing condition that would come to bear his name. The following year, a European doctor named Dr. Alois J. Beuren noticed the same thing. In Europe, the condition would come to bear his name as well.

Williams worked at Greenlane until 1964, when he was offered a job at the Mayo Clinic in the United States. He accepted but never showed up for work, heading instead to London. Later, the Mayo Clinic offered him another post and again he accepted but this time, he disappeared entirely, leaving a suitcase checked in a London luggage office that was never claimed. No one could explain what happened to him.

Gloria and her family would not hear of the mysterious Dr. Williams, his odd disappearance, or the strange condition he described, for another twenty-five years.

{chapter 2}
MESMERIZING MUSIC

G loria played with blocks in front of a one-way mirror. When she glanced up from her haphazard pile—which was often, because blocks couldn't hold her interest for very long—she saw only her own reflection: the face that had grown scrawny, the smile that had grown toothy, the eyes exaggerated and puffy, as if with sleep.

What Gloria did not see was the small army of experts watching her every move on the other side of that mirror. Sometimes they were psychologists, sometimes therapists, sometimes medical doctors, all searching for clues in her every move and gesture. Sylvia took Gloria to the Dade County Developmental Evaluation Clinic in downtown Miami every week for more than a year. They hoped for answers, or at least a clue as to what Gloria's future might hold.

The experts watched Gloria play alone, noted how she flitted from toy to toy to toy, so easily distracted. They watched her with other children; she seemed utterly indifferent. And they watched her with adults, when she was totally transformed. She touched them gently, held their hands, hugged them. She reveled in their attentions, almost anxious to share whatever she had, so eager to please, so eager to be loved. It was not typical behavior.

31

The experts discussed, debated, argued, hypothesized, and finally shared their conclusions with Howard and Sylvia. There are three levels of mental retardation, Howard and Sylvia were told. The highest is "educable," where the person retains some higher cognitive function and can actually learn concepts and abstractions. Such people have a stab at living a fairly independent life. The next level is "trainable," where the person can be taught to perform simple tasks correctly, but can hope for little more. Such people would always need close supervision. The last level is "profound," and it means that there is little hope for the kind of life and fulfillment that Howard and Sylvia so wanted for Gloria.

Gloria, they were told, fell into that first group. The highest group. Gloria was educable.

In a bizarre way, the news made Howard almost giddy. He felt a strange rush of pride, followed closely by the more familiar pangs of anguish. He couldn't cry, so he laughed. "Do you mean my daughter is at the top of the class?" he joked.

Bernie went to the school closest to their house, a lovely Spanish-style building of white stucco and red tile. Only "normal" children went there. When Gloria entered public school in 1959, Sylvia drove her to farther-away Miami, to a school equipped for the handicapped. It was a low-slung, ranch-style building of red brick, surrounded by garden plots where children grew flowers and fruits and vegetables. The gentle tending of these gardens, Howard and Sylvia would soon discover, was about as rigorous as Gloria's academic instruction would get. The school was Dade Elementary, and Gloria's classroom was filled with children who couldn't speak or walk well, who had this or that syndrome, who needed "special education." They did not interact with the school's regular kids. They were kept on their own. Away.

There were eighteen little desks in the classroom that Gloria would attend for the next several years. It was a cheerful room, festooned with brightly colored construction paper and the ABCs and a dusty green chalkboard, much like you'd find in any elementary school classroom. But its students made it entirely different.

The range of disability there was daunting. Some of the children were hyperactive. Others were prone to roughhousing. Others, like Gloria, couldn't pay attention for very long. The teacher was a woman of remarkable patience and iron will named Josephine Shappee. Josephine wore glasses, had fluffy brown hair, a soft face, and an extremely gentle voice, and she amazed Sylvia. Josephine never seemed to lose her cool. She had a tender way with them that inspired confidence; when Gloria lost interest in her work and started to wander off—which was often—Josephine calmly but firmly steered her back to her desk and her schoolwork. When Gloria grew upset because the other kids were being too loud or pushing too hard or being too ornery, Josephine helped her learn how to handle conflict. When Gloria needed hugs and affection, Josephine provided an abundant supply.

How do you do it? Sylvia once asked her.

They rest me, Josephine said.

Sylvia told Josephine everything she could think of about Gloria's diagnosis and problems, about how she was so responsive to music and loved nursery rhymes, about how she could carry a tune and adored singing. Josephine assured her that there were plenty of songs and nursery rhymes in her classroom, and then gave Sylvia an idea: if Gloria loves music so much, why don't you get her into a church choir? That would almost certainly be a great boon to her development.

Howard and Sylvia had never considered such a thing before. The idea seemed ripe with possibility, and with peril: What if Gloria simply couldn't do it? What if she failed? Singing the proper thing, at the proper time . . . was Gloria really capable of that?

They adapted the church choir idea—they were, after all, Jewish—and Sylvia gingerly approached the choir director at their synagogue. There were terse nods and tight smiles and it quickly became clear that Gloria would never sing a note with that group. The word "no" was never uttered, but Sylvia's request faded into the ether and was never mentioned by the choir director again.

They were learning not to expect much from the world where Gloria was concerned. For all the kindness and inspiration of Gloria's teacher, Howard and Sylvia came to understand that drawing and painting were the main activities for special education students in Miami's public schools, and lessons often revolved around whatever holiday was next: Halloween, Thanksgiving, Christmas. Howard and Sylvia were inundated with cut-and-paste jack-o-lanterns, and turkeys traced from Gloria's stubby fingers, which they dutifully hung on the refrigerator as they waited for her to learn to write her name, read a book, add one plus one. Gloria was proud to see her work displayed for all to see; Howard and Sylvia couldn't help but notice that she couldn't manage to color inside the lines.

The school did try to teach academics with the state-of-the-art educational technology of the early 1960s—mimeographed worksheets. Worksheets for reading. Worksheets for math. Worksheets designed for kids who knew how to hold pencils, who could manipulate them well enough to make something approaching writing, and who could, most vitally, read. Gloria's ear for languages was so keen and her vocabulary was so strong, it seemed like reading shouldn't have been a struggle. It was. She could not comprehend how black squiggles on a white page represented the rich and varied sounds she heard. To her it was all just a collection of crazy lines, random and indecipherable, signifying nothing.

Arithmetic was an even grimmer endeavor. The worksheets covered rudimentary mathematics—two plus two equals four,

four plus four equals eight. But numerals confounded her. What, exactly, did they represent? What *were* they? She couldn't wrap her mind around "four," or how it differed from "five," or how that differed from "six." The concepts of more and less—the bedrocks behind addition and subtraction—were gibberish to her. As Howard and Sylvia watched her struggle, they felt an icy fear for the future: Gloria might never be able to handle her own money, pay her own bills, balance her own checkbook. What would become of her? Who would look out for her after they were gone?

Gloria took the academic frustration in stride. She truly loved school. She thrived on the company of other people, and school was, above all, a social experience for a very social child. Her attention usually centered on adults—teacher Josephine may well have been the most hugged person in the state of Florida—but a sweet boy with Down syndrome became her best friend and shadow, answering her toothy grins with grins of his own. He loved to draw and paint, and Gloria attempted to do the same, working contentedly beside him. She loved story time and singing—especially singing—and even when she was sick, she wanted to go to school.

Most of the kids in regular classes had never seen handicapped students before. They didn't understand what was wrong with them, why they were sent off to a room all by themselves, why they were different. There were always a few children who excelled at cruelty, and they teased Gloria for the funny way she walked and for the thickness of her glasses. They called her a retard, an ugly duckling, and laughed. One Easter, two neighborhood girls, both Catholic, accused her of killing God because she was a Jew.

Such unkindness struck Gloria like a physical blow. She couldn't comprehend all of the names that were being hurled at her, but she understood the emotional tone of the attacks perfectly. It hurt so terribly: why were they being so mean, when all she wanted to do was be friends? She burned to respond to their taunts, but didn't know how; she would stiffen and shake in silent torment and fury, her face growing red until tears spilled down her cheeks. That only sparked more derision. Once, an enraged Bernie witnessed one of these sessions and bloodied the nose of a ringleader. But Bernie couldn't be there all of the time, and bloodying noses wasn't a long-term solution to the problem. Howard and Sylvia thought they had become intimate with every subtle shade of heartache, but this was an even deeper agony. How to possibly explain the savage, conformity-enforcing cruelty of children to someone as sweet and uncomplicated as Gloria? They stammered and stumbled as they tried, but came out with various versions of "sticks and stones may break my bones, but names will never hurt me."

They knew better. And so did Gloria. She was strangely, acutely sensitive to the colors of their moods. When Sylvia was putting on a brave face, trying to dismiss the bullies, Gloria saw past her bravado and seized on the underlying sadness. "Are you OK, Mom?" Gloria would ask, studying Sylvia closely.

Gloria retreated into the refuge of her family. Her grandmother had moved in and became a best friend: "Bubbie," as she was called in Yiddish, taught her to manipulate a needle and thread well enough to embroider, and soon the house was awash in needlework. Gloria learned to knit and pearl a straight line, but never quite mastered how to make anything curve; Howard and Sylvia wound up with a large collection of extremely long, multicolored scarves, which were just what they needed in Miami's relentless humidity. The sound of grandmother and granddaughter singing Yiddish songs as they knitted ever-longer scarves in the tropical Coral Gables heat became one of Howard's most prized memories: one of Gloria's favorites was the playful song "Der Rebbe Elimelech," a celebration of music calling for the fiddler to step up and strut his stuff. *"Az der Rebbe Elimelech iz gevaren zei-er freilich, Iz gevaren zei-er freilich, Elimelech. . . ."*

When Howard and Sylvia were trying to make peace with the prospect that Gloria might never be able to read or write well, she surprised them—something she'd be doing quite often in the future. A young psychologist had developed a new reading method for special education students that stressed phonics in small, incremental steps; teacher Josephine welcomed the psychologist into her classroom, and Gloria became part of this special project in fourth grade. She began poring over workbooks every afternoon, and something in her head clicked. She could comprehend the sounds, and their relation to the black squiggles on the page. By the end of the year her reading had improved dramatically—by several grade levels—and she could identify numbers well enough to attempt Go Fish at the kitchen table with the rest of her family. When the fates conspired in her favor and she won the game, Bernie or Howard or Sylvia would still have to inform her of her victory; even with a fistful of winning cards, she had little concept of which number was greater than another.

Every little step felt like a major battle, a major victory. They just didn't know what to expect from Gloria.

Gloria did not thrive in the tropical heat. She was scrawny and small, her hair perpetually in pigtails, suffering the usual array of childhood illnesses complicated by an odd reaction to the humidity: it often left her unable to breathe. Howard and Sylvia had to catch their own breath as she was hooked up to an oxygen tank. She had trouble with her teeth and developed a primal fear of the dentist, getting so hysterical that the dentist refused to treat her unless she was sedated.

Many of the youngsters in the neighborhood outgrew her. Bernie began to be embarrassed by her in front of his friends. Sylvia had to arrange outings with disabled kids from her class so she'd have playmates—perhaps the first playdates. But that didn't impress Gloria much; what brought her the greatest joy were the affections of adults like her grandparents, aunts, and uncles; and most any kind of music. It was hard to explain, exactly. Gloria seemed physically hungry for music. It riveted her, focused her, excited her. Every child deserved an outlet they enjoyed, Sylvia figured; there had to be a way to teach her something about it. There had to be something she could learn.

Sylvia was rattled by the bad choir director experience but hit the phones nonetheless, finally finding a woman who taught piano to the blind. Someone experienced working with handicapped people. Someone who could work around barriers. Sylvia delivered Gloria to the teacher's house and watched tiny Gloria slide onto the bench of a grand piano; her pigtails stuck out, and she suddenly looked like a little bird lost at sea. The teacher proceeded to speak in arcane musical concepts—chords, progressions, scales, octaves—leaving Gloria completely bewildered. *Every Good Boy Does Fine are the notes on the lines. FACE are the notes between the lines. There are whole notes, half notes, quarter notes, eighth notes. . . .* Sylvia drove her unsmiling daughter home, sure they wouldn't be going back for a second lesson.

A new round of phone sleuthing led Sylvia to a piano teacher with a master's degree in psychology. Someone with a concept of what might be going on inside Gloria's mind, who could be sensitive about how to reach her. Jan Call had never worked with special needs children before, but agreed to give it a try.

Jan was a pretty, bubbly blonde whose South Florida friendliness quickly put Gloria at ease. Jan was able to forego music theory's abstraction and concentrate on the concrete; she let Gloria plunk her way along the keyboard, listening to the tones, without mentioning octaves or inversions or eighths. Ultimately, Jan helped Gloria compose a melody all her own. Gloria's song was sweet and simple; "Meranda," Gloria called it. Gloria had aptitude, if not exactly talent, Jan believed, and said it was just a matter of time until Gloria learned to read music. Jan started slipping in formal music theory during Gloria's keyboard explorations; Sylvia saw the familiar glaze creep across Gloria's face, but was relieved when Jan didn't push it too hard. Over two years with Jan, the scrawny, pigtailed Gloria grew bigger and her tiny hands grew more confident on the keyboard. Sylvia had hope that Gloria might really find a pleasurable outlet in music. That seemed the most anyone could hope for.

♪   ♪   ♪

Gloria went through puberty early. There were no uncomfortable talks about why it happened or what exactly it all meant; Gloria was simply told it was something that happened to women, and that she was becoming a woman now. She liked the idea of that.

As her eleventh birthday approached, Sylvia decided the perfect present would be a more formal musical instrument. But it couldn't be a bowed or stringed instrument; she really didn't have the coordination to manipulate those. Ideally, it would be something related to the keyboard, to draw on her years of piano lessons. If electronic keyboards had been invented back then, Gloria surely would have gotten one.

Sylvia was poking around the music store in the Gables when a half-size accordion caught her eye. One designed for kids. It was candy-apple red with bright white keys and buttons. If she had understood that it required pumping of bellows and pushing of buttons and playing of keys all at the same time, she surely wouldn't have bought one for Gloria; but she knew nothing about how an accordion is actually played. She simply thought, why not? It had a keyboard. It seemed like a logical progression.

Gloria's birthday parties were populated primarily by adults, not children. There was the newly found cousin Irving Lenhoff—once a prizefighter—who taught Gloria how to jump with both legs in the air and attempt snazzy self-defense moves. Howard's parents were there, as were an array of aunts, uncles, and cousins. Sylvia had ordered an elegantly decorated chocolate cake from the fancy bakery in the Gables, and there were candles and piles of brightly wrapped presents and choruses of "Happy Birthday."

The accordion was in the biggest box. Gloria carefully unwrapped it, opened the case, and immediately slipped the straps over her shoulders. It was awkward; the frozen joint in her right elbow forced her to hold it at an odd angle. But she ran her fingers over the keys, began pumping the bellows and fingering the buttons. Slowly, surely, she picked out melodies with her right hand on the keyboard, and with some internal calculus unknown to Howard and Sylvia, figured out which chords went along with them and pressed those chord buttons with her left hand. "You Are My Sunshine," "Oh, Susanna," "Clementine," "My Country 'Tis of Thee" were among the songs in her repertoire. Howard and Sylvia were flabbergasted. Nobody in the family played the accordion. Nobody knew what the heck to do with it. How had she figured it out? How had she managed to coordinate so many different movements? Maybe, they thought, she saw it on *The Lawrence Welk Show*. They whispered to each other: they had better find an accordion teacher. Fast.

The music store put them in touch with Mrs. Alzarez, a Cuban refugee who lived past the cemetery. Mrs. Alzarez assigned Gloria pieces to learn and books to study, which didn't go over well; Gloria seemed more interested in trying to speak to Mrs. Alzarez in Spanish than in learning the assignments. Gloria stopped after about ten lessons, but remained interested in the instrument on her own terms, playing it every day and picking out new tunes that she heard on the radio. Howard and Sylvia found it interesting, and strange.

When a Jewish girl turns twelve, she becomes a "daughter of the commandments." She is responsible for herself under Jewish law, obligated to follow the commandments in the first five books of Moses, and able to participate in all aspects of Jewish life. The bat mitzvah ceremony formally marks this rite of passage; at services on one of the holy days, the child is called up to the Torah to recite a blessing, lead the congregation in prayers, and sing traditional chants. "Today, I am a woman," girls often say. The joy of a bat mitzvah day is supposed to equal the joy of a wedding day.

As Gloria's twelfth birthday approached, Howard and Sylvia had a big decision to make. They dearly wanted Gloria to experience a bat mitzvah and all its magic, but they weren't sure she could do it. There was so much involved; not just memorizing the prayers and chants, but doing them at the right time and in the right order, while staying calm and collected in front of all those people. It required a level of attention and concentration that they weren't sure Gloria possessed. To make it even harder, the Lenhoffs belonged to one of the largest synagogues in Miami. Developmentally disabled boys and girls simply weren't bat mitzvahed there in 1967.

But someone, they decided, had to be the first. Gloria would pass into womanhood the way other Jewish girls had before her.

Rabbi Landau was understanding and supportive. In Conservative Jewish circles, bat mitzvahs usually happen on Saturday mornings, the Sabbath day, when large crowds have been known to pack the temple. On one hand, Howard and Sylvia thought that would be a wonderful way to celebrate; but on the other, they were plagued by visions of Gloria losing her place, forgetting her lines, and being overwhelmed and embarrassed in front of everyone they knew. So they came up with a compromise: Gloria would be bat mitzvahed on a Saturday evening in a small side chapel, rather than on a Saturday morning in the cavernous main temple.

Mr. Louis Gadon, a thin, frail man with a gravelly voice, became Gloria's coach. One of the chants she would sing in Hebrew would be chapter 6 of the Song of Songs—a story of fierce love told by a woman who makes no apologies for her passions. The Song of Songs is seen as an allegory for the relationship between God and the people of Israel.

Mr. Gadon didn't change his ways for Gloria. He did what he

always did to teach the soon-to-be bar and bat mitzvahs the prayers and chants: he recorded himself carefully enunciating each word and singing in a scratchy falsetto, then gave the recording to the child to study and memorize. Gloria listened to it every day for months, reciting it over and over, line by line.

When the day finally came, Howard and Sylvia were far more nervous than Gloria. The change in her seemed enormous: the scrawny little girl with pigtails had become a chubby young lady with stylishly close-cropped hair. Immaculate white gloves lent her an air of polish and sophistication, and she wore a pretty dress of white and blue, the colors of Israel.

The chapel was festooned with flowers and filled with nearly one hundred people. On the altar, with the rabbi, Gloria began chanting the Song of Songs. Howard and Sylvia held their breath. In a sweet, soft voice, she sang in Hebrew and announced to the world she had arrived into Jewish adulthood:

> Where has your beloved gone, O fairest of women?
> Where has your beloved turned, that we may seek him with you?
> My beloved has gone down to his garden, to the flower beds of baisam, to pasture in the gardens, and to gather lilies.
> I am my beloved's, and my beloved is mine, who pastures among the lilies.
> You are as beautiful as Tirzah, comely as Jerusalem, as over-awing as the most distinguished.
> Turn your eyes away from me, for they dazzle me. . . . Who is she that appears like the dawn, as beautiful as the moon, as bright as the sun . . . ?

Throughout the chapel, eyes welled. It was perfect. Gloria hit every note, enunciated every syllable, kept perfect tempo. There was a moment of stunned silence as she finished; the girl who hadn't shown much promise for anything had done something difficult and had moved her audience to tears. It was a powerful moment, and she knew it. She felt the emotion in the room, and it electrified her.

Up to this moment, Gloria's life had been lived behind a wall. Her disabilities separated her from others, kept her at a distance, made real connections difficult. But, with this ceremony, with this song, it felt like walls had come tumbling down, like she had broken through an awesome barrier and entered a wondrous place.

"Oh Lord, I thank you, my parents and grandparents, my teachers, relatives, and friends, for helping me to reach and to celebrate my bat mitzvah," she read from a speech her parents had prepared. "I am happy and proud to become a young Jewish adult, and to accept more of the responsibilities of our people. Please, oh God, help me to spread happiness and understanding in the way that I best can—through music, through song, and through doing mitzvahs. Amen."

Afterward, in the synagogue's reception hall, was the ceremony of the candles. The most beloved people in Gloria's life lit them, one by one: schoolteacher Josephine Shappee, music teacher Jan Call, grandmother Bubbie, brother Bernie, and many more until finally, Howard and Sylvia lit one themselves. "It is enough to say that this is one of the happiest days of their lives," the rabbi said as the candles flared.

Afterward, Gloria picked up her new, full-size accordion and played the "Anniversary Waltz" for Howard's parents, who were celebrating their forty-fourth wedding anniversary. As the proud grandparents danced to their granddaughter's music, Howard and Sylvia were overcome with emotion. How had Gloria learned to play the "Anniversary Waltz" on the accordion? Something was going on here. Something very strange. Something very special.

"Gloria's bat mitzvah was one of the most moving and thrilling experiences of my entire rabbinate," Rabbi Sol Landau soon wrote to the Lenhoffs. "She has indebted us all by her musical gift, her warmth of personality, and excellence of performance."

The rabbi nominated Gloria for a new award bestowed by Dade County upon people who exceed expectations. Gloria was among the charter group of winners.

♪ ♪ ♪

Gloria soon discovered opera on Saturday afternoon radio, and fell madly in love. Its crazy passions, soaring arias, and exotic languages mesmerized her. She watched operas on public TV, raided her parents' record collection, and played them on the stereo until she knew them by heart. She was enthralled by their convoluted plots of devotion and despair, one wilder than the next: *Madame Butterfly was so in love with her American husband that she waited for him for years, pining, aching, raising the son he had never seen. When he finally returned to her—with an American wife!—she made the ultimate sacrifice, giving up her son so he could go to America with his father. Madame Butterfly was so devastated, she killed herself.... Prince Tamino, lost in the forest, was pursued by a serpent and fainted from fatigue. Three ladies, all attendants of the queen, saved him and killed the serpent with their lances. Each lady fell in love with the prince, and plotted to possess him.* She seemed to inhabit these epic and sweeping and fantastic stories, feeling their exaggerated emotions as if they were her own.

Howard and Sylvia were surprised at how easily she memorized pieces in Italian and German, mimicking the pronunciation, intonation, and emotional phrasing of the divas on the records. She sang along with the highest soprano parts; those, to her, were the most beautiful. She couldn't translate most of the words she was singing, but she seemed to understand the emotions— yearning, fury, loss—and did her best to channel them. *Tosca, Il Trovatore, Turandot, Otello, La Bohème, Aida, Le Nozze di Figaro*—she loved them all and couldn't get enough.

Sylvia was helping put together a benefit for Goucher College when Ann Wilson's résumé fell into her lap. Ann had also gone to Goucher and was a professional concert singer, willing to sing at a benefit for Goucher's scholarship fund. Ann had performed in Paris, London, Hamburg, and elsewhere in Europe, specializing in lieder and other art songs.

All that was well and good, but when Sylvia got to the part in

Ann's résumé about how the singer had done "diversional music therapy" in New York City hospitals and prisons, she jolted to attention. Any woman who could walk into a prison and coax incarcerated audiences to song had to be special. Surely, if Ann could help them find joy in music, she could help Gloria, too.

Ann was a woman of regal bearing, small and powerful, in the way of many professional singers. She was partial to Mozart and Schubert and lived in a near-Gothic mansion in one of Miami's toniest neighborhoods. She had no experience with handicapped students, but loved teaching; her mission, as she saw it, was "vocal rejuvenation," pulling voices back from the brink of damage and helping their owners find control and discipline. She considered that her specialty.

Gloria had been singing along with technically punishing operatic pieces for some time, and at Gloria's first lesson with Ann, she launched into one of those impossible arias. Ann winced. Gloria was a soprano, Ann felt, but her voice stretched and strained and pushed and pinched, and was well on the way to damage. What are we going to do about this? Ann thought.

Ann sang Gloria a snippet of Mozart's delicate song, "Come, Lovely May," and asked Gloria to sing it back to her. Gloria opened her mouth and sang in a high, thin voice; Ann was impressed by how completely Gloria remembered what she'd heard. It turned out that Gloria had to hear a piece of music only once or twice to remember it in its entirety; and Gloria could imitate whatever Ann played on the piano almost effortlessly. But she concluded that Gloria couldn't create music, or interpret it, from inside herself. Gloria was extremely musical, profoundly musical, but not in a way Ann had ever encountered. Ann would later say that she had no experience with that kind of talent—or handicap.

Ann went in search of Gloria's real voice. Not the voice she expertly copied from radio or record, but her real, true, core voice. Her goal was to teach Gloria to seamlessly blend that core with her head voice—the highest notes she could reach—and teach her to sing well. It was Ann's belief that very few pop singers knew how to sing well. Frank Sinatra was an exception— he had a real voice and learned how to use it properly—but these youngsters, all they knew how to do was yell. Gloria would do exercises to strengthen her voice and learn to use her larynx properly. Gloria would learn control and discipline, things that didn't come easily to any singer, and she would still be singing "Come, Lovely May" perfectly forty years after she learned it.

In Gloria's two years under Ann's tutelage, her voice grew truer and stronger. But teacher and student separated when Howard accepted a four-month post teaching marine biology at the University of Hawaii, then a yearlong stint at the Weizmann Institute of Science in Israel in 1968. Gloria wasn't fond of the sea or sand in Hawaii, but she learned many songs in the exceptionally musical Hawaiian language; and she wound up at a fine school for the disabled in Israel, where she learned her first Sephardic Yemenite songs, as well as traditional folk music and a phrase that came in handy with her pushy classmates: *"B'lee yadaim!"* Literally, "without hands," or more colloquially, "Keep your paws off me!" It's a phrase she would use for the rest of her life.

Howard soon accepted his first full-fledged academic job in Southern California. He would become associate dean of biological sciences and full professor at the fledgling University of California at Irvine, in bucolic and conservative Orange County, about an hour south of Los Angeles. Sylvia became an administrator at the university. The family moved to a roomy house with a backyard pool on Robin Hood Lane in quietly suburban Costa Mesa, where the weather was perfect most of the year, the long scarves Gloria knitted remained obsolete, and the search for good music teachers for Gloria began anew.

{*chapter 3*}

EXPOSITION

Gone was the salty, sultry, sticky air of Miami; the Lenhoffs tried to get used to cool ocean breezes and the scent of sweet orange blossoms mingling with manure in what was then agricultural Orange County, California. Gone also were the hustle and bustle and diversity and resources of Miami; the Lenhoffs tried to adjust to the calm and quiet and homogeneousness of a new and growing area. Gloria had a hard time saying good-bye to her old friends but was excited by the prospect of meeting a whole new set of people. Their house was on a cul-de-sac, with a brick path leading through the green lawn to the cozy front porch. It was 1969, and bulldozers and cranes were still carving out a campus at new UC Irvine. It was surrounded by cow pastures and orange groves, and students could peek out windows and watch hooves kick up dust from distant cattle roundups. Life was going to be much different than what the Lenhoffs were used to on the East Coast. If it was hard to find the kind of things Gloria needed in Florida, it seemed like it would be ten times harder here.

Howard and Sylvia started their search for a new music teacher for Gloria by calling the Mardan Center of Educational Therapy in Irvine, a nonprofit special education school that was just a few years old. They were referred to music therapist Dick Kuykendall.

Dick had taught at a private school for the autistic and spent almost a dozen years at Fairview State Hospital, a state mental institution in Orange County. He was a pianist and singer whose mission was to use music to change behavior. He believed music could help Gloria learn to stay on task, improve her muscle coordination, and learn how to stop changing the subject abruptly in conversations. His philosophy was that students don't learn, they "catch"; if the teacher models good behaviors, the students will catch them. Eventually. It's a matter of perseverance and repetition.

At their first session together, Gloria sang Dick some Italian art songs she had learned with Ann. He was impressed. Her voice was not strong, but her pitch was perfect, her breathing seemed natural and her phrasing was easy and unhurried. She doesn't need music therapy, he said. She needs music *lessons*.

And for the next several years, that's what she got. Dick gave her exercises to strengthen her voice. She wanted to sing high soprano pieces, but he heard a lot of strain in her voice and encouraged her to develop her lower registers. In his opinion, she was an alto, not a soprano. He taught her songs in Italian, French, English, and German. She grew particularly fond of "Oh Divine Redeemer" by Charles Gounod. Over their years together, he worked on focusing her attention on the work at hand, until she could sit still and concentrate on music for the entire hour they spent together each week. He considered that a big success.

When Dick moved to Michigan to pursue his own studies years later, Howard and Sylvia's search for vocal teachers began anew, again. An ad in UCI's student newspaper led them to a pre-law student who soon realized there wasn't much she could teach Gloria. Why don't you just send Gloria to *my* teacher? the student said. That's how they found Barbara Hasty, a lecturer in voice at UCI, who would become Gloria's mentor for the next decade and beyond.

Barbara was from Dallas and, by the oddest of coincidences, had gone to college with Dick Kuykendall. She had never worked with a cognitively disabled student before, but as a colleague of Howard's on the UCI staff, she felt it was a matter of professional courtesy to see if she could work with Gloria. Barbara had a master's degree in voice from the University of Southern California and had done the professional circuit, singing at festivals and touring Europe until she married a minister and had children. Then, her income was the only one they could rely on, so she began teaching at the college level. Barbara's philosophy was plain and simple: anyone could be taught to sing. Their success, she believed, depended far more on their passion than on their gift, far more on how much they wanted to sing than on how naturally talented they were. She had seen determination and a love of music best talent again and again, and felt it was her job to tease the best out of whatever a student had to offer. She agreed on this point with Dr. Shinichi Suzuki, who developed a successful method to teach music to young children: everyone has natural ability, and ability grows when it is nurtured. The beauty of a voice, Barbara believed, is mostly learned, not made.

Gloria and Barbara met in a studio at UCI, and Barbara asked Gloria to sing. *Far above average,* Barbara thought as she listened. Gloria's breathing seemed intuitive. Her phrasing seemed natural. And she seemed to understand the proper style in which to sing a particular song. If anything was lacking, Barbara decided, it was in the area of technique: Gloria carried a lot of tension in the neck area, around the larynx, and they would have to work on that. Barbara asked Gloria to do physical exercises to relax and loosen up her shoulders.

Don't sing with the chin jutting up and out, Barbara would say. That stretches the muscles in the larynx and adds even more tension to the voice. Tuck that chin in! They developed a routine: Gloria brought a tape recorder to their lessons. Barbara gave advice, demonstrations, and sang Gloria a new aria or art song.

Gloria listened to it again and again over the next week; and she knew the new song by the next lesson. Barbara began to feel that Gloria could sing anything, in any language. Gloria picked up on foreign languages so easily that Barbara couldn't help but feel Gloria must have had some sort of acquaintance with them in the past. Once she gave Gloria the first six pages of a Mozart aria to learn in Italian; Barbara didn't bother with the last two pages because the piece turned florid and show-offy, as if someone besides Mozart had finished it. When Gloria came back the next week, she knew the entire aria, including the pages Barbara hadn't bothered to sing.

How on earth did you do that? a stunned Barbara asked.

We have a recording at home and I just listened to it, Gloria explained. Barbara found it uncanny. Gloria's musical memory was so precise it was almost spooky.

It was as if Gloria had lived another life and had knowledge of music, Barbara said. Nearly a decade would come to pass between the time Gloria first learned Strauss's ethereal "Morgen!" and the day Barbara pulled it back out and asked her to sing it again. Gloria had instant recall and sang it flawlessly, as if she had been working on it the day before. *"Und morgen wird die Sonne wider schienen"*—"And tomorrow the sun will shine again."

I probably couldn't have done that myself, Barbara thought. After nearly a decade, I might remember the music, but I'd surely forget the German. In her entire career, Barbara would never have another student like Gloria. Gloria was from a different part of the stratosphere. After every lesson with Gloria, Barbara came away with a new sense of what life was all about.

Howard and Sylvia ferreted out a series of accordion teachers to tutor Gloria from ads in the student newspaper, including people with delightful names like Marc Moreels and Siggie Kukier, who would remain her friends for the rest of her life. During their investigations, Howard and Sylvia discovered the growing phenomenon of "summer camp." In California they came across surfing camps, swimming camps, horseback-riding camps, baseball camps, bible camps—and they started looking around for a camp for Gloria. It would have to be especially for the mentally handicapped, and they hoped to find one geared to music and Jewish youth through their local synagogue.

When they came up empty-handed, they turned to local Jewish community centers. Nothing. They expanded their search to include synagogues and centers in nearby San Diego and Los Angeles. Still nothing. They started searching throughout California and then the nation; no religious classes, no summer camps, no retreats geared to the Jewish handicapped anywhere. Nothing at all. Most every program for handicapped kids was run by a Christian church—usually a fundamentalist Christian church—where great emphasis was put on praising Christ. In the end, this is where Gloria went. She came back singing about Jesus, and Howard and Sylvia decided that was just fine. The Christians showed Gloria warmth and respect, gave her an opportunity to grow, to learn, to laugh, to experience some joy. But it bothered Howard: why couldn't the Jewish community do the same thing?

Howard became fixated on trying to fathom why. In Israel there were wonderful programs for handicapped Jews. But in America—where, outside of Israel, the largest Jewish population lived—there was nothing. Did this attitude come from the Bible, which implied that, to make offerings and prayers, you must be physically perfect? Was it because Jews held learning in such high regard that those who couldn't achieve in study were seen as somehow less human? Was it because the disabled made people too painfully aware of the tenuousness of their own lives? He didn't expect to find an answer, but he hoped that by probing, by asking uncomfortable questions, something might change. He expected more from his community of faith, and made it a point to prick its conscience at every opportunity. He harangued rabbis, wrote scolding letters to newspapers, started getting a reputation as a pest. He considered himself as extremely determined, intending to change things that needed to be changed. Eventually summer camps run by Conservative Jewish synagogues began accepting mentally retarded kids, but by then, Gloria was too old and didn't need them anymore.

In Orange County, as in Florida, Gloria attended special education classes. But she would proudly say that she sang in a chorus with regular kids at Corona del Mar High, and even enrolled in choral classes at Orange Coast College, where she earned all As. When she finished public school at age twenty-one, she was handed a diploma. It didn't mean that she possessed a body of knowledge; it was more like a receipt from the public school system, saying it had done all it could do, and now someone else must take over.

Howard and Sylvia were at a loss. What now?

College, of course, was an impossibility. It would be wonderful if she could find work using her musical abilities, but meaningful jobs for the mentally disabled were virtually nonexistent. Howard and Sylvia asked around and found a widespread perception that retarded people were only capable of work with what they called the "Four Fs": food (washing dishes); flowers (gardening and yard work); folding (napkins in restaurants or sheets as chambermaids); and filth (custodial work). Handicapped people who wanted to work were expected to toil in "sheltered workshops" with others of their kind—not with regular people.

Sheltered workshops were usually found in cavernous buildings in nondescript industrial parks. They were filled with disabled people who spent their days stuffing envelopes, collating reams of paper, or sliding plastic forks and knives into the plastic packets served with airline dinners. It was unskilled, repetitive, and often mind-numbing work. The government provided the bulk of funding for these well-intentioned programs, which began in the 1950s and 1960s so disabled people had a reason to get out of bed in the morning and a way to earn some money of their own. Defenders said sheltered workshops were a valuable transitional step before entering the competitive work force; detractors called them sweatshops. Workers earned less than minimum wage, and the jobs were hopelessly dead-ended.

But what choice was there? Gloria, like every disabled person on the cusp of adulthood, needed and deserved a focus for her life, something that gave it meaning. She needed to be surrounded by people. So Howard and Gloria sent her to do the only thing she could do: take a job in a "sheltered workshop" and embrace one of the Four Fs.

Gloria started clocking in at a workshop in Fountain Valley, California. Her mission, for a time, was to assemble first aid kits in white metal boxes emblazoned with red crosses. Her workstation was in a vast room where she'd grab a box, place bandages carefully inside, then insert instant ice packs and a first aid instruction book. Her production rate wasn't high because she was far more interested in people than in packing; but she learned how to punch in and out with a time card and took coffee breaks with her coworkers. "We do all sorts of contracts for businesses," she would proudly say, and Howard and Sylvia came to conclude it was well run. Gloria enjoyed the companionship of the other workers and was glad to have something to do.

She did get into some trouble for talking instead of working, as talking now tied up her hands. She learned some sign language from watching a deaf colleague: "Very, very happy!" she'd say with fingers flying. "No cry. Smiles. We're friends, right?" Howard and Sylvia thought it uncanny that her facility with languages spilled over into sign language as well. She learned to sign "Back to work" when breaks were over, and more and more of those breaks were spent with Bill MacDonald, a handsome young man with dark hair, warm eyes, and an engaging smile. They wrapped their arms around each other at the lunch table. Gloria leaned her head dreamily on his shoulder. When lunch was over, they exchanged little kisses on the lips. The romance never progressed further; Howard and Sylvia didn't think Gloria had any idea romances ever progressed any further. She didn't ask any questions, and they didn't feel the need to give her more information. She was in love, she said. She was happy. And so long as someone with a watchful eye always had the lovebirds in full view, Howard and Sylvia were happy, too.

Gloria religiously attended her voice and accordion lessons, and Howard prodded the powers-that-be at the workshop to find work for her that involved music. There wasn't much to be found. She did a brief stint in the nursery at a fitness center, watching children while their parents exercised, but it didn't go well; too much responsibility for Gloria, and not enough adult supervision. She loved the kids, though, and was soon working part-time as a volunteer aide at a preschool where the teachers kept a much closer eye on her. Gloria tied children's shoes in her own unusual way, pushed them on swings, helped them wash their hands at snack time, put their mats out at nap time. She handed out lunches and shushed the whiners who didn't want any vegetables, telling them to eat because it's good for them. She slipped smocks over their heads when it was time for finger painting and oooh'd and ahhh'd at their colorful creations. She rumpled hair, doled out hugs and kisses, and said, "Love ya!" to all the children and teachers.

But the highlight for Gloria was sitting beneath a shady tree, all the children gathered at her feet, and playing the accordion for song time. The kids would belt out the "ABC Song" at the top of their lungs; Gloria's operatic soprano would soar above, warbling "Now I know my ABCs, next time won't you sing with me?" in a positively comical manner. The children would grow uncharacteristically quiet as she sang "Somewhere over the Rainbow." They were very much like her: yearning to be loved and hugged, and reveling in music.

There were mishaps. Gloria fell prey to the illnesses sweeping the students, which put great strain on her voice. And learning to travel to and from her jobs was a logistical ordeal: At first, Sylvia rode the buses with her, showing her where to get on and off and transfer, while Howard followed in the car. Then they let her try it on her own, while both Howard and Sylvia followed in the car. Eventually, Gloria learned to travel on her own. Once, though, she got lost in an unfamiliar city and had to ask a policeman to take her home. Howard and Sylvia's worry for her never completely disappeared, and at the end of the day, they strained to hear the sounds indicating she had gotten off the bus safely and was walking home: they could hear her singing all the way.

Gloria worked long enough to qualify for Social Security benefits on her own. Now a working woman with a small income — Howard always felt that the compensation paid to Gloria was laughable — Gloria developed a taste for shopping. Clothes shopping, food shopping, it didn't matter to her; it was the ambiance of stores, the opportunity to chat with salespeople, the thrill of paying for things herself, even if she never was sure she got correct change, that pleased her so much. One of the largest and most glitzy malls in the nation was just a few miles from her house: she wandered in and out of boutiques in Costa Mesa's fashionable South Coast Plaza, admiring pricey jewels and trendy fashions, never letting Sylvia out of her sight. Gloria couldn't afford to be separated from her mother because she would be utterly lost; malls were indecipherable mazes, and if she wound up alone she would never find her way back to where she started.

There was one item in particular that had caught Gloria's fancy: makeup. It was the era of blue and green eye shadow, of hot pink lipstick and crimson rouge, of thick mascara and jet-black eyeliner. Gloria bought baskets of the stuff in every imaginable hue, and spent hours experimenting before the mirror. When she emerged, Sylvia was often startled or amused: "Gloria, you look like a clown!" Sylvia would say. "I do not," Gloria would retort. "I like wearing makeup. I know how to put it on right."

In her off hours, Gloria spent time with books. While Howard was busy researching the plight of the Ethiopian Jews, which had begun to consume him, Gloria perused her shelves lined with fairy tales of sleeping beauties and Cinderellas; books explaining how babies grow with full-color pictures of eggs fertilizing, blastocysts dividing, and fetuses sucking their thumbs in the womb; and volume after volume on opera. There were act-by-act synopses of the great works, complete guides to learning and loving them, biographies of her favorite opera stars like Beverly Sills and Maria Callas. She could often be seen on the bus going to one job or the other with volumes tucked under her arm, and she liked to ask new mothers if they had a natural birth or a Cesarean. There were a few singing gigs here and there, including one at a local retirement community, which paid her thirty dollars, but it clearly wasn't a living. She saved up the money to buy a television set because she wanted to watch her favorite shows—the operas aired on PBS—on her own TV bought with her own money.

Howard and Sylvia had always known that Gloria's disability would dictate the rest of their lives, but now it became visceral. She was grown up, but she was a child, would always be a child, needing and wanting to be led, cared for, protected, praised. Bernie was grown and gone, out of college, starting his own life; but Gloria would never leave. Someday, Howard and Sylvia would be the ones leaving her. And then what? Who would take care of Gloria the way they did? They couldn't ask Bernie to assume that kind of a burden. Gloria had worked long enough at the sheltered workshop to qualify for Social Security benefits of some three hundred dollars a month, but that couldn't support her. For Howard and Sylvia, it wasn't the certainty of their own deaths that they feared; it was what would happen to Gloria after they were gone.

Howard started writing. He channeled his complicated emotions into a book, *Conception to Birth: Human Reproduction, Genetics, and Development*, explaining the male and female reproductive systems and all that can go wrong when sperm and egg meet and begin to divide.

"The statistics indicate that from 2 to 5 percent of children born in the United States have varying degrees of physical and mental handicaps," he wrote. "They also show that parents who are educated have fewer children with handicaps than those with less education. It is my wish, and my major incentive for writing this book, that readers will be sufficiently knowledgeable that they will have even fewer children with either congenital or hereditary birth defects.

"Nonetheless . . . a number of you will have a handicapped child. What if it is you? How are you going to handle it knowing that the rest of your life is going to be very different from the life that you as a college student had planned? Will the mental strain be too much? Will you feel guilty that something that you did caused the handicap? Will you feel that you have been unfairly selected to bear this burden? Will you institutionalize the child? Can you afford it? If the child does manage to survive and adjust until adulthood, how will you provide for the child's future, especially after you are dead?

"There are no easy answers. I can only offer prospective parents of handicapped children a word of hope, based upon my own experiences as the father of a mentally and physically handicapped daughter. I refer to my oldest child, Gloria, to whom I have dedicated this book. Gloria . . . was born prematurely with the use of forceps following the obstetrician's decision to break the amniotic sac. At first we did not believe that

Gloria had any handicap although we did suspect that every-thing was not just right.

"I will not go into the details of Gloria's early years, but they were not easy on her and on the rest of the family. All we learned from the physicians was that Gloria was short for her age, tested as educable mentally retarded, and had a few physical defects such as a heart murmur, unusual gait, and a partially 'frozen' joint in the elbow of her right arm. But something happened around her 13th birthday when she participated in her Jewish confirmation ceremony, her 'Bat Mitzvah.' To avoid 'embarrassment,' we arranged to have the ceremony in a small chapel, and we hoped for the best. To the amazement of all present, as part of the ceremony, Gloria sang from memory in a beautiful soprano voice a number of ancient Hebrew melodies, including the melodious Song of Songs of King Solomon. In addition, she picked up her accordion, a gift given to her just two weeks beforehand, and proceeded to play, without any instruction, a number of songs.

"From that moment outwards, our lives changed. Why? Because Gloria broke us of the stereotype that mentally handicapped individuals are devoid of talent. She proved that she did have strong untapped talents, and that with a little help, she could not only enrich her own life, but the lives of most people that she touches. As a parent, I began to think more about her and less about myself."

Howard's book was the text for the popular course he taught at UCI, From Conception to Birth, enrolling five hundred students a semester and requiring the largest lecture hall on campus. It always concluded the same stirring way: with Gloria singing to a packed lecture hall of undergraduates, who exploded into applause and gave her a standing ovation. Gloria adored the praise, the heat, the light. Many of the students were moved to write letters to Howard and Gloria, saying how much they enjoyed her performance and how inspiring she was. Gloria kept all of them and loved to page through them. One letter stood out:

It was from a young man who was struggling with drug addiction. He saw how Gloria had struggled against enormous odds to make so much of her life, while he had every advantage a person could hope for and was throwing it all away. He vowed to pull himself together and use his talents. If Gloria could excel, he wrote, maybe he could, too.

Just one hundred miles away, Sandy Miller was having a heck of a time. Her daughter, Amanda, was so small the doctors said she must have been born prematurely—even though Sandy was certain she had been pregnant for the standard amount of time. When Amanda screamed inconsolably and failed to grow, the doctors said there must be a problem with her blood vessels. When Amanda failed to walk by age one, the doctors told Sandy to calm down and lighten up; not all children develop at the same pace and she should just be patient. When Amanda finally took her first steps at twenty-one months—and then, to Sandy's shock, started running three days later—the doctors concluded that Sandy was obviously an overprotective mother who had been holding her baby back the whole time.

It was maddening. Up until then, Sandy had believed everything the doctors told her. But she knew she wasn't an overprotective mother, and she knew Amanda's development wasn't normal. Even after the family moved from New Mexico to California, the doctors still didn't believe her when she insisted something was wrong; because Sandy was a physical therapist, she expected everything to go by the book, she was told. Everything, of course, doesn't go by the book.

It was at one of those standard checkups that the doctors started to understand what Sandy had been saying for years. The doctor burst into the examining room and beamed at Amanda, saying, You have new shoes on, don't you? Aren't you cute!

Amanda stared at him, impassively. Hmmm, the doctor thought. Amanda was two and a half. A girl that age should be responding to such prompts, showing off her shoes, acting coy and cute. Amanda did nothing.

The doctor sent Amanda to UCLA for tests. The experts called Sandy in and pulled a massive book off the shelf; *Human Malformations*, its spine read. It was thicker than a phone book. They opened it and pointed to a small article with fuzzy black-and-white photographs: "Williams syndrome," it said.

And there, in *Human Malformations*, the mother found her child. Everything was there—from the elfin nose to the slowness to walk, from the inconsolable screaming to the developmental delays. There was no known cause, and no known cure.

Yes, Sandy said. This is my Amanda.

Amanda was almost three. Sandy then knew for sure that the developmental delays would not be something her daughter would outgrow. Amanda was mildly to moderately mentally retarded.

Sandy searched for more information about Williams syndrome, but there was precious little to be found. The latest theory was that it was somehow triggered by high concentrations of calcium in the bloodstream. Sandy discovered that, in England, there was a new group called the Infantile Hypercalcaemia Foundation—their name for Williams—and she sent away for information. Soon Sandy received flyers and brochures and became the North American information clearinghouse on the condition. She urged doctors to get her the names of other Williams families in Southern California, and soon they all were meeting regularly in San Diego, offering one another advice and support. Sometimes doctors would attend these gatherings, too, to discuss the latest science regarding Williams. Organizing events for a dozen far-flung families wasn't easy, but Sandy was adamant about doing it; if she could prevent a single parent from going through the uncertainty and frustration and hurt that she went through, her efforts were worth it.

As parents unloaded their fears and hopes, there was a story Sandy loved to tell. It was about how Amanda, from the second she could stand up, would hang on the piano. She wasn't even tall enough to see the keyboard. She'd stick her arms up high over her head until she felt the keys. She wouldn't pound away indiscriminately, as so many toddlers did; instead, she picked out perfect, harmonious notes.

Sally Meersman laughed at the coincidence. Sally lived in Fountain Valley, a city in Orange County just a few miles from Costa Mesa, and her daughter, Mary, was diagnosed with Williams at age two. Mary was more withdrawn than other Williams children, but Mary would snap to attention whenever she heard music. She'd listen with the most comically intense look on her face. Mesmerized. Ah, well. All kids love music, don't they? she thought.

{*chapter 4*}
HI HOPES

Not far away in Orange County, teacher Doris Walker was assigned a challenge: invent a music class for special education students. She played piano, but had never taught music before, and could find little literature to guide her; so she decided to just play simple songs and let the kids sing along. After all, every kid loves to sing.

This is in the key of G, or C, or D, she'd offhandedly explain as she began a song.

Paul Kuehn was one of her students at Hope School. Blind and almost completely nonverbal, he had a history of sitting in the back of other classrooms and rocking, occasionally banging cans together. One day, Walker sat down to play a song and mumbled, Which key did I play this in last week? A voice piped up from the back of the room: The key of G, Paul said.

Those were the first and only words Paul had ever spoken in class. Walker came to understand that her profoundly disabled students could also be profoundly musical: Paul's rocking had been to the beat of songs he heard on the radio. He soon started vocal lessons, and slowly, surely, his voice grew in depth and character. He made his debut at a parent-teacher meeting, where he crooned the love-struck ballad Sir Lancelot sings to Lady Guenevere in *Camelot*—"If Ever I Would Leave You"—with so much emotion that some listeners lost their breath.

Paul stuck with the singing lessons and when a donated drum set landed in the classroom, he took to it immediately. His voice grew into a rich, deep baritone, and he created drum arrangements for the songs Walker played in class. At first, they played only single-chord songs like "Row, Row, Row Your Boat." Emboldened, they tried two-chord songs, and then graduated to three-chord songs, the bread and butter of rock 'n' roll. Other disabled people showed musical ability as well, and in 1972, there was enough critical mass to form a band. The first band made up entirely of mentally disabled musicians, as far as they knew. Hi Hopes, it was called.

They started small, playing only for sympathetic and forgiving audiences at PTA meetings and elementary schools. Audiences fully expected to be embarrassed for the musicians, but after hearing Paul belt out "The Impossible Dream," attitudes changed. Hi Hopes graduated to gigs at churches, fairs, and Elks and Kiwanis club meetings all over Orange County.

The Lenhoffs heard about the band through a friend. They planned a big bash for Gloria's thirtieth birthday—including a formal recital in the living room—and invited the Hi Hopes bandleader to attend.

Folding chairs were packed between the sofas in the Lenhoffs' living room as neighbors gathered to hear Gloria sing Mozart and Schubert. As soon as Gloria opened her mouth and that powerful soprano burst forth, Walker knew she had found Hi Hopes' newest member. A savant, without question, she thought. Delighted, Gloria agreed to join Hi Hopes, unaware how profoundly the world would open up to her.

As the newest member of Hi Hopes, Gloria felt like she was no longer alone. There were others just like her, with profound abilities and disabilities, making joyous music. Finally, she was getting to do the thing she loved more than anything in the world: sing to people, live in the flesh, intimately, face-to-face. The old saw about performers living for the crackle of applause was literal truth for Gloria; singing, and the voltage shooting through the audience when the song was done, were vital.

Gloria adored her new friends. She thought Paul was a wonderful drummer; he, too, had perfect pitch and could shake your rib cage with his rendition of "The Star-Spangled Banner." He had an astounding ability to name the artist who recorded any song you could think of, along with the precise year it was recorded. They worked out a duet of the "Hawaiian Wedding Song," and it was great fun to sing it with him.

She would also come to fuss over Gary Ahearn's skill on keyboards, banjo, guitar, and just about any other instrument he touched.

But Gloria found a special friendship with singer Lori Reyes, "the little girl with the big voice." Lori, an alto, was a fearless performer with a flair for the dramatic, just like Gloria. Lori was outgoing and curious and loved being around people, just like Gloria. And she bore an uncanny resemblance to Gloria: they both had puffy eyes, wide mouths, and upturned noses. They both had to wear thick glasses to correct poor vision. They were both quite small. Everyone used to joke that they were long-lost sisters. The band became like a family.

Word spread that Hi Hopes was a troupe of "idiot savants." Its tour schedule would expand to a breakneck 180 performances a year from one coast to another—one every other day. Guest numbers in Las Vegas and at the Grand Ole Opry in Nashville; performances at fund-raisers for the mentally impaired in Washington, DC. Eunice Kennedy Shriver was so moved by Gloria's "Ave Maria" that she flew Gloria to Massachusetts to sing at the dedication of a new center for the disabled. Ted Kennedy adjusted her microphone.

Gloria became something of a celebrity. "A show-stopping voice, clear and soaring," one article said. "A talented young woman of warmth and vivacity," said another. Flash bulbs popped and cameras rolled; Hi Hopes was featured in newspapers, on national television, in *Time* and *People* magazines. Gloria and the others began learning answers to the questions reporters always asked. "It's the best thing that God gave me," Gloria would say about music. "Some people don't realize what handicapped people can do. . . . I don't know why we have this. I just know we do, and people like us." The applause was thunderous.

Howard and Sylvia had to step back and process it all. Singing for audiences was like a magic potion that transformed their daughter; it allowed Gloria to sidestep her shortcomings and connect directly with people on the virtue of her strengths. She was happy. But for all the exhilaration, the band was time-consuming and exhausting. The logistics of getting Gloria to practices and gigs were demanding, and Howard was finding himself pulled in too many directions as he became ever more active in the grassroots movement to convince Israel to give a permanent home to the Ethiopian Jews. The endless phone calls, meetings, letter-writing campaigns, and media interviews sometimes left him feeling drained. Everyone had to sacrifice: Hi Hopes families and staff found themselves canceling personal events to keep band engagements. Howard also longed to see more opportunity for the band members. Why did talented but handicapped people have so few opportunities? Why couldn't they make music a vocation and go into the world with a marketable skill? It seemed obvious that Gloria and the other Hi Hopes members should be able to make a contribution—and a humble living—through music. Some could play regularly for people in nursing homes and preschools as actual consultants or employees, rather than as volunteers on a hit-or-miss basis, as they did now. Others could perform at piano bars, in hotels, at recitals, or at conferences for the handicapped.

Howard became president of the Hi Hopes board of governors and together they pursued that vision: a residential university of fine arts for handicapped people. Soon, however, the strong personalities and differing visions of Howard and Walker began to clash. Howard worried that Gloria was ceasing to grow musically. Walker felt that Howard wanted too great an emphasis on Gloria. Tension was high.

♪   ♪   ♪

Arlene Alda couldn't put down the March 2, 1987, edition of *Time* magazine. "The idiot savant has a long tradition in the U.S., much of it as victim," the story read. "A typical 19th century savant, Tom Bethune was sightless and barely able to grunt monosyllables. But he had the ability to play complicated classical piano pieces by ear, and promoters exhibited him in vaudeville as an amusing freak.

"Since that time, savants—retarded and autistic people who have inexplicable gifts, usually in art, mathematics and music—have been the objects of diversion and exploitation. But at a unique institution called Hope University in Anaheim, Calif., they are being trained to reveal their surprising gifts and develop self-confidence."

Arlene was an accomplished still photographer who could plug into innocence and imagination with such ease that she wrote many successful children's books. But there was also a time, not so long ago, when music was her entire world. She played the clarinet, won a Fulbright scholarship to study music in Europe, and joined the Houston Symphony Orchestra as assistant first clarinetist under the direction of legendary conductor Leopold Stokowski. She gave up a promising music career in 1957 to marry a struggling young actor named Alan Alda.

Even though she became a photographer and writer, music was still a big part of her life, and the prospect of these musical savants was riveting. What were they like? She must know more. But the story didn't seem like it would lend itself well to still photography or even to prose; hearing the music these savants made would be vital to a full appreciation of their world. The story, Arlene decided, must be told on film.

Of course, she had absolutely no experience with film. But she didn't let that stop her. She contacted Dr. James Maas, chair of Cornell University's psychology department. Arlene and James had had an unlikely first meeting: every year during the December holidays, the Maas family vacationed at the same resort on St. John in the US Virgin Islands; and every year, the Alda family did the same. Maas first met Alan Alda on the tennis courts, and they all became friends.

James Maas's love of film began in the early 1960s, when he worked summers for Eastman Kodak in New York. When he became a professor at Cornell, he merged his love for film with his love of teaching, and made films on sleep disorders, drunk driving, perception, psychiatry, child development, educational methods, and outstanding teachers. He showed the films to his introductory psychology lecture classes, which swelled to seventeen hundred students and became what he believed were the largest lecture classes in the world. His films wound up on PBS; the BBC; the Canadian Broadcasting Corporation; and Dutch, Danish, and Swedish national television.

Arlene called James and urged him to read the *Time* magazine piece. He was instantly smitten. They wasted no time calling Hi Hopes with the idea of a documentary and drumming up funding. Just a few weeks later, first-time director Arlene Alda, photographer/producer James Maas, and three Cornell students, shouldering heavy lighting and sound equipment, climbed aboard a plane to Orange County. They would shoot film, not video, and the documentary would air nationally on PBS.

The budget was small, so they checked into a very basic motel then headed straight to the two cramped rooms in the Anaheim strip mall where Hi Hopes worked . . . and where things were quickly unraveling.

To Arlene and James's surprise, exclusivity became an issue. There was talk of cost and rights and dollar figures that were beyond the reach of a public television documentary's budget. After some tense exchanges, the crew packed up and left, disappointed and fearing that they had wasted thousands of dollars.

Arlene, James, and the crew retreated to their motel. They were depressed, making plans to leave. Then they spoke to Howard. He said all was not lost: they could, if they wanted, film Gloria, and probably at least one other band member, Paul Kuehn. Gloria and Paul had incredible stories. They'd be great subjects for a film.

James and Arlene thanked him, but it wasn't what they had planned. Focus on only one or two people? That seemed so narrow. They envisioned a documentary about the spectacular, singular school they had read about in the magazines. They wanted to capture the Hi Hopes band in concert, to scan the faces of the audience during standing ovations, to glimpse behind the scenes into the lives of a cast of amazing, disabled performers. Dropping the school entirely and focusing on just one or two people seemed so thin in comparison.

Necessity is the mother of invention, Plato said. The more Arlene and James thought about it, the more they started to see possibilities in focusing on just one person. Narrowing the story could lend great depth. Instead of a whole band, there would be one singer; instead of a half-dozen lives, there would be one. The theme was still about how talent can thrive despite disability; perhaps this would let them tell the same story in an even richer way.

They had come all this way and spent all this money. What the heck. It was worth a try.

The next day, Arlene, James, and the crew went to the Lenhoffs' house to meet Gloria and consider their options. The first time Arlene heard Gloria sing, she was transfixed. She doesn't read music, Arlene thought. She has to learn everything by ear and memorize it. The music. The lyrics—in a foreign language. And then she has to solve the problems every musician faces: phrasing, emotion, understanding. It was an awesome task and Gloria did it with great feeling; but at the same time, she didn't seem to know which piece to do next and seemed dependent on the direction her father gave. Gloria was a revelation, and Arlene felt a powerful connection to a kindred, musical spirit.

Maas was struck by her stage presence and her ease before the camera. She was completely comfortable, not affected or self-conscious at all. A natural. They became convinced that this was the way to go.

Howard knew that, by becoming the focus of this documentary, Gloria would be persona non grata at Hi Hopes and would no longer be singing with the group. She would miss the friends who had become her extended family over the past five years, that he knew. But he also knew that Gloria's story should be told and trusted that something just as good, if not better, would be waiting around the next corner.

Arlene, James, and the crew practically moved into the Lenhoffs' house and became Gloria's shadows for the next eight days. What a lovely home you have, Arlene told the Lenhoffs, then proceeded to have the crew rearrange furniture and lights and pictures to fit production needs. Arlene and James followed Gloria to her job at the preschool. They followed her to her job at the workshop. They filmed her at synagogue chanting evening prayers, at her voice lessons, in the mall, putting on her makeup, helping around the house. They shot hours of interviews with Howard and Sylvia as well as with Gloria, trying to capture the reality of her life. When the family erupted in spontaneous song, the crew scrambled to get their cameras, careful to keep Arlene's husband out of the shot.

At first, James was confused. Where, exactly, was Gloria's mental retardation? Savants were usually terribly introverted, isolated, noncommunicative, devoid of social graces; but the woman he saw through the lens of his camera, though quiet, was warm and engaging, asking after people's children and parents, remembering everyone's name. It took him a while to figure it out; as he watched her meet more and more new people, he realized that the conversation was often remarkably the same. Gloria had a social script that she had somehow learned, and she could perform it flawlessly. She would ask the same questions with the same emotional tones, answer questions with almost prerecorded answers. It was odd. Something he had never seen before.

But watching Gloria go through the world, there was no mistaking her genuine love for other people. James and Arlene saw how she looked at her mother and father; they saw her face after singing Puccini; they watched as she doted on children; marveled as she spoke in sign language with her deaf coworker. Arlene and James found themselves falling in love with Gloria.

When Howard started talking about the future, their hearts ached for him. Howard spoke clearly, candidly, about his deepest fear: he and Sylvia weren't going to be around forever, and they wouldn't be there to make sure Gloria got to her singing lessons, had a chance to perform, got the love and attention she required. For more than thirty years they had attended to her every need, but they knew that, someday, they'd have to find a place for her to start life on her own. It was a constant pressure, a constant strain, like an ache that never, ever eased. They hadn't figured it out yet, but they knew they had to.

One of the last days of filming was the most poignant. Howard was teaching his From Conception to Birth class to a large lecture hall full of undergraduates at UCI. Statistically speaking, he told them, 5 percent of their offspring—or thirty-five children, if each student in the room had two kids—would suffer birth defects.

What would you do? he asked them. How would you handle it? Without revealing who she was, Howard summoned Gloria onto the dais. Ask her to sing a song in any language, Howard said. Italian! Japanese! Spanish! the students shouted. Each time, Gloria obliged. Then she sang the ardent aria "Voi che sapete" from *Le Nozze di Figaro*, "*Voi che sapete che cosa e amor, Donne, vedete s'io l'ho nel cor*" — "You who know what love is, Ladies, see if I have it in my heart." The students went wild.

"Gloria, I understand your mother is here today," Howard said. Gloria locked eyes with Sylvia and said, "Hi, Mom," which brought more applause.

Then Howard said, "Gloria, I understand your father is here today, too." Gloria made a big show of scanning the lecture hall, squinting into the distance and turning her head to and fro, until her gaze landed back on Howard. Then she smiled a tremendous smile, her voice softened, and she gave him a hug. "Hi, Dad," she cooed. The camera crew wiped away tears, the students exploded into applause, and Gloria turned her face to the crowd with that look of absolute, utter bliss.

At that moment, Arlene and James knew they had captured what they were looking for. "In everybody there's something — what you have to do is find out what it is, treasure it, nurture it," James said. "There are so many religious lessons, moral lessons, human lessons there."

Arlene felt the same way. "It raised my consciousness tremendously about the possibility of human endeavor," she said.

Arlene and James went into the editing room. Arlene loved watching the footage and shaping the story, but even a lightning-fast edit of twelve weeks felt agonizingly slow to her. She much preferred the shoot-and-see world of still pictures. When searching for a title, they settled on something Sylvia had suggested: *Bravo, Gloria!*

Bravo, Gloria! went first into competition in film festivals. It won several awards, including the Silver Medal at New York's International Film and TV Festival. Howard was excited. When its premiere on public television was scheduled for 10 PM on Sunday, May 1, 1988—when, Howard thought, few people would actually be able to see it—he tried not to be disappointed. TV stations just don't care much about stories about the handicapped, he told himself. That was nothing new. He planned a premiere party at their house, inviting friends, popping popcorn, and settling in to watch in the ever-present folding chairs. Gloria parked herself close to the television and beamed as her face appeared on screen and everyone erupted in cheers.

"I want to have a good life. I don't want my life to go down the drain," the TV Gloria said. "I want people to realize that I have a handicap but I want them to know that I'm a special person."

Gloria giggled as she saw herself shopping in the mall, packing first aid kits at the workshop, working with children at the preschool. "They like to be loved and wanted and hugged a lot," the TV Gloria said. "They like me to play with them. It's really fun. I like being with them."

When Sylvia and Howard's faces popped on the screen, Gloria lit up. "That's you, Mom!" she said. "Look at Daddy!"

As students leaped to their feet in the final lecture hall scene, the image froze on Gloria's face, wide-eyed and blissful, in the midst of a deep bow. The scene in the living room mimicked the one on the TV screen precisely: people leapt to their feet, and Gloria gave them a deep and appreciative bow.

You're a national TV star now, Howard told her. From coast to coast, from the Canadian border to the Mexican border, millions of people have heard you sing. You're helping to change the way they think about disabled people.

Gloria smiled. It was quite a prospect.

It didn't take long for the Lenhoffs' phone to ring. It was a colleague, saying he'd seen *Bravo, Gloria!* and thought it was very good. But the colleague was confused: Why didn't you mention that Gloria had Williams syndrome? he asked.

Williams syndrome? Howard asked. What the heck is Williams syndrome?

It's a rare condition and it's obviously what Gloria has, the colleague explained. She looks like a pixie who tumbled out of a storybook. Elfin face, upturned nose, sharp chin, broad mouth — all classic signs of Williams syndrome. She's mentally retarded, hopeless when it comes to numbers, struggles with gross and fine motor coordination, walks with an awkward gait, has bad vision. But that warm personality and social grace — all classic signs of Williams.

But what *is* Williams syndrome? Howard asked again.

As best as anyone could tell, Williams syndrome was a mistake on the genetic or biochemical level, he was told. No one had figured out exactly how it happened yet. Scientists speculated that it might have something to do with an overproduction of calcium while the fetus was developing, but that was just one theory. It probably happened once every twenty thousand to fifty thousand births, but it was hard to say. So many Williams people weren't diagnosed, because so many doctors had never heard of it. Just as James and Arlene and Howard and Sylvia had never heard of it.

Howard listened, only mildly interested, to the description. Yes, it certainly sounded like Gloria, Howard agreed. But really. Wasn't this just academic? Gloria was in her thirties. Who needed a diagnosis at this late stage of the game? They had struggled long and hard to give Gloria a good life, and they felt like they'd done a good job. Gloria was a classically trained lyric soprano. She held two jobs. She had people who loved her and places to sing and was the subject of a nationally broadcast documentary film. She was happy. What difference could a diagnosis possibly make now?

{chapter 5}

THE VEIL LIFTS

Sally Meersman was thrilled to learn that the new Williams celebrity lived so close to her in Orange County—and she was determined to add the Lenhoffs to the ever-growing Williams family. She and her daughter, Mary, lived less than fifteen minutes away from the Lenhoffs, and Mary had always been so mesmerized by music, ever since she was a tiny baby. Mary would just love to hear Gloria sing, live and in person.

The little group of Williams parents that Sally helped organize six years earlier had done quite a bit of growing up: it had blossomed into the Williams Syndrome Association, a nonprofit with more than one thousand members from coast to coast. It was now a clearinghouse for the latest information on Williams, from how to handle educational issues to the latest scientific research. Sally was the membership director, and she wanted the Lenhoffs to be members. She called them and urged them to come to a Williams picnic slated for Mile Square Park in nearby Fountain Valley on Saturday. It's so wonderful to meet other Williams families, Sally assured them. You'll love it! Please come.

A picnic? The Lenhoffs weren't sure. Gloria wasn't a child anymore. She didn't play outside. And they certainly didn't need the succor and support of other parents going through the trials and tribulations they'd already gone through.

But Howard's curiosity gnawed gently at him. Maybe, probably, most likely, Gloria did have Williams syndrome. What were other kids with Williams like? It could be interesting to see. Saturday turned out to be a brilliant Southern California day, the sunshine so warm and crisp that it made every last blade of grass seem to stand out in hypersharp focus. So Howard packed up Gloria's accordion, stopped to buy a New York cheesecake, and headed for Mile Square Park.

The park was an urban oasis of glistening lakes, wooded hiking trails, and emerald golf courses. The Williams families were to gather in the picnic area, so he and Gloria made their way across a great expanse of green lawn, Howard lugging Gloria's accordion in one hand and the cheesecake in the other.

Several picnics were in full swing, with barbecues blazing and children dashing about. Howard squinted, trying to figure out which group was the one he was looking for. A tiny girl ran by: Gloria as a toddler. He stopped nearly dead in his tracks. Then there were more apparitions: Gloria as a schoolgirl. Gloria as a teenager. Gloria as a young adult. Everywhere he looked, he saw his daughter.

He had found the Williams picnic, and it was a revelation. He couldn't believe how much the Williams people resembled one another—that upturned nose, those puffy eyes, that pointy chin. They could be brothers and sisters, he thought.

The kids rushed at him and Gloria with the zeal of running backs and chattered with the charm of talk-show hosts. "I saw you on TV!" "How are you?" "Where do you live?" "What's your name?" "Do you have a favorite TV show?" Many of the children had received countless warnings about not talking to strangers, but they simply couldn't help themselves. Howard had always considered Gloria quite verbal, considering her disabilities, but some of these kids were truly a world beyond. How extraordinarily friendly and curious and loquacious these children are, Howard thought.

Howard spent the rest of the afternoon huddled with the parents, listening in stunned disbelief as they described their children: Miserable babies. Slow to walk. Slow to talk. Prone to heart troubles, digestion troubles, sight troubles, teeth troubles. Expresses himself well. Great sensitivity to others' feelings. Has a good memory for birthdays and obscure trivia. Poor problem-solving skills. Never forgets a face. Fascinated by foreign languages. Can't draw or do math. Problem with depth perception. Hyperacute hearing. Trouble tying shoes, fastening buttons, cutting with a knife, concentrating for more than a few minutes at a time.

Howard reeled. It was as if Gloria's life was being recited by complete and total strangers, as if their words could be coming directly from his mouth. Gloria, meanwhile, attended to the younger kids with the authority and expertise she had honed at the preschool. They wanted to know what was in the big black case, and when she told them it was an accordion, they demanded that she play. Howard watched the children closely as she obliged; they deserted swings and stopped their games and swarmed around her like bees, buzzing, probing, investigating. Most had never seen an accordion before, so they closely examined its keys, buttons, and bellows, nearly pressing their faces against the instrument, much as Gloria had done to Howard's guitar strings when she was a baby. "It's loud!" some laughed, covering their ears, but not one left. They sang along to "Old MacDonald," "Eensy Weensy Spider," and other songs Howard suggested, greedily mooing and oinking and cock-a-doodle-dooing, happy to listen for as long as Gloria was happy to play. When it was time to go, Howard felt like he had been shot through with adrenaline.

At home, he tried to explain to Sylvia. It was one of the most eerie afternoons of his life. Like seeing yourself on *This Is Your*

Life. Something strange happened at Mile Square Park. Something amazing was going on. They absolutely, positively, had to delve deeper into the literature on Williams syndrome.

There wasn't a great deal written about Williams, but Howard devoured everything he could find. What he read made the hair stand up on the back of his neck.

The very first mention of the condition was in the 1961 paper by New Zealand cardiologist J. C. P. Williams, followed about a year later by German cardiologist Alois J. Beuren. They described children who shared a strange, similar narrowing of the aorta, the main artery leading from the heart. That narrowing prevented the heart valve from opening and closing properly, obstructing blood flow.

Howard remembered Gloria's heart problems as a baby. The visit to a New York cardiologist when she was four months old. The way her tiny body lit up when she was examined by the powerful rays of a fluoroscope.

The children looked strikingly alike, the researchers wrote, even though they weren't related. They were elfin, small and fine-boned with upturned noses, sharp chins, and haunting eyes that often had white, lacy, snowflake patterns in the irises.

Howard saw Gloria and the other children in the park, looking like an extended elfin family.

In 1964 researchers G. von Arnim and P. Engel described the psychological characteristics of the syndrome, and were struck by the children's "friendly and loquacious" personalities and their "unusual command of language." They also noted, in passing, that the children enjoyed music.

Howard saw the buzzing hive of children in the park, and heard Gloria sing.

Mental retardation was the most common feature of the syn-

drome, next to the elfin face, the researchers said. Some 95 percent of Williams people had IQ scores in the moderate to mildly
mentally retarded range. Gloria was firmly in the middle, with an
IQ of fifty-five. Most were in special education classes, and their
academic performance in math and problem solving lagged far
behind their peers'. Even in adulthood, a vast majority had only
basic skills in reading, writing, and math. As a result, adults with
Williams syndrome either lived with their parents or in super-
vised group homes.

For Howard, a familiar shudder. What would happen to
Gloria after he and Sylvia were gone?

Some of the most intriguing research on Williams syndrome was
being done just one hundred miles south of the Lenhoffs' home,
in the labs of the Salk Institute for Biological Studies in San
Diego.

One evening in the mid-1980s, Ursula Bellugi was in her lab
long after the sun had sunk into the blue Pacific just beyond the
Salk's windows. Bellugi's fascination had long been the biological
foundations of language — where it resided in the brain, how the
systems worked. She and her colleagues made their mark by
proving that American Sign Language is a formal, genuine language, complete with its own grammar and syntax, and processed
by the same parts of the brain that handle spoken language in
hearing people. Her work led to the discovery that the left hemi-
sphere of the human brain becomes specialized for languages,
whether spoken or signed, which she calls "a striking demonstra-
tion of neuronal plasticity."

It was late when Bellugi's phone rang. The caller introduced
herself as Nancy Verougstraete. She lived nearby in San Diego
and had just finished reading a magazine piece by Noam
Chomsky on the biological foundations of language that mentioned Bellugi's work.

If you really want to investigate the neurobiological underpinnings of language, Verougstraete said, you must meet my daughter.

Oh? said Bellugi.

Verougstraete explained that her daughter, Wendy, had a condition called Williams syndrome. Wendy was fourteen, with an IQ of about fifty, and she read and wrote at the first-grade level. But she had the personality of a cheerleader and the language of a poet.

"You are looking at a professional book writer," a cheerful Wendy would later say. "My books will be filled with drama, action, and excitement. And everyone will want to read them. I am going to write books, page after page, stack after stack. I'm going to start on Monday."

Curious, Bellugi agreed to meet Wendy, and her fascination with Williams began.

"I was puzzled," Bellugi told the *New York Times*. "She had a very unusual profile. Her grammar was complex and without error. Her word use was rich, but general cognition and problem solving were very impaired. She had been placed in a school for the mentally retarded but her teachers did not know how to deal with her. I looked around for information on cognitive abilities of Williams syndrome but very little was known."

Science had long taken for granted that language and reasoning were inextricably linked. Those who were the most agile with language, the most expressive and witty, were usually the most intelligent as well. But Williams syndrome seemed to shatter that view of intelligence. It promised to help tease those processes apart.

Bellugi decided that, first, she needed to understand which traits set Williams people apart from people with other syndromes. She started by matching Williams children with Down syndrome children for gender, age, and IQ.

The differences in ability were stunning. When she asked a Down teen to name all the animals he could think of, the teen said, "Dog, cat, fish, bird, fish." When she asked a Williams teen, she was astounded by the answer: "Brontosaurus, tyranadon, brontosaurus rex, dinosaur, elephant, dog, cat, lion, baby hippopotamus, ibex, whale, bull, yak, zebra, puppy, kitten, tiger, koala, dragon."

When she asked a Williams teen to draw an elephant, the drawing was unrecognizable: One large circle—the body—with some squiggles representing the head over here, an eye over there, the trunk elsewhere still. The mouth was a separate circle, floating freely off in space.

Almost as if the teen knew how indecipherable his picture was, he tried to make up for it with words.

"What an elephant is, it is one of the animals," the teen said. "And what an elephant does, it lives in the jungle. It can also live in the zoo. And what it has, it has long, gray ears, fan ears, ears that can blow in the wind. It has a long trunk that can pick up grass or pick up hay. If they're in a bad mood, it can be terrible. If the elephant gets mad, it could stomp; it could charge. Sometimes elephants can charge. They have big long tusks. They can damage a car. It could be dangerous. When they're in a pinch, when they're in a bad mood, it can be terrible. You don't want an elephant as a pet. You want a cat or a dog or a bird."

In addition to having amazing vocabularies, Williams people could be incredibly expressive, Bellugi found. She showed the teens a panel of three drawings, and asked them to make up a story to go along with it. In the first drawing, a little boy and his dog are looking delightedly at a frog in a jar. In the second drawing, the boy and the dog are asleep on the bed, and the frog is escaping from the jar. In the third drawing, the boy and the dog look forlornly at the empty jar.

The Down syndrome teen, age eighteen, IQ fifty-five, made up this story: "The frog is in the jar. The jar is on the floor. The jar on the floor. That's it. The stool is broke. The clothes is laying there."

The Williams syndrome teen, age seventeen, IQ fifty, invented this story: "Once upon a time when it was dark at night, the boy had a frog. The boy was looking at the frog, sitting on the chair, on the table, and the dog was looking through, looking up to the frog in a jar. That night he slept and slept for a long time, the dog did. But the frog was not gonna go to sleep. The frog went out from the jar. And when the frog went out, the boy and the dog were still sleeping. Next morning it was beautiful in the morning. It was bright, and the sun was nice and warm. Then suddenly when he opened his eyes, he looked at the jar and then suddenly the frog was not there. The jar was empty. There was no frog to be found."

The Williams teens were also incredibly animated when telling their stories. They altered vocal pitch, volume, word length, and rhythm to enhance the story's emotional tone, Bellugi wrote. Sometimes they spiced things up to engage the audience, exclaiming, "And suddenly, *splash*!" "BOOM!" and "Gadzooks!"

But as Bellugi continued to study Williams people, she discovered a strange disconnect between the richness of their language and their understanding of it. Once, a girl emptied a glass of milk into the sink and said, "I'll have to evacuate it." Once, a child gave Bellugi a drawing and said, "Here, Doc, this is in remembrance of you." Once, a Williams person explained how she wound up in regular high school classes, saying, "They said that I had the genius of a regular student." Bees didn't "fly away from" or "leave" the beehive, they "aborted" it. These word choices could be considered syntactically correct, but semantically they were just a little off the mark, Bellugi said.

In contrast to all this verbal richness, Williams people had a stunningly deep deficit in spatial thinking. Bellugi and her colleagues showed them a series of slanted lines and asked them to pick out the lines that matched. They couldn't even do the practice items correctly.

To test their understanding of spatial relationships,

researchers showed Williams kids a large pitcher of water, then poured the water into several smaller bowls and asked if there was more water, or less. Of course, water transferred from one container to another retains the same volume, regardless of the container's shape. It's a concept that taps into general cognitive ability and is usually mastered early. The Williams kids however, could not comprehend it. To them, it seemed ludicrous that those little bottles held as much water as that giant container.

Bellugi also found that Williams people tend to process visual information piecemeal, rather than as a whole. She showed the kids a drawing of a big letter *D*—which was made up of many tiny letter *Y*s—and asked them to copy it. Williams kids drew many tiny *Y*s, completely ignoring the large *D* shape. Down kids drew the big *D*, ignoring the fact that it was made up of tiny *Y*s. It became clear that Williams people saw the trees, while Down people saw the forest. And it became clear that reasoning and verbal ability were not as closely linked as people once believed.

Williams syndrome was fast becoming Bellugi's lifework. Struggling to understand the spatial deficits, she found that Williams people had another mysterious and incongruous "island of ability": facial recognition. Parent after parent told stories about how their children never forgot a face; one even spotted the Italian model Fabio strolling down a city street. Who the heck is Fabio?! the mother said.

It didn't seem like this should be the case. It stood to reason that people who couldn't match patterns or draw coherent pictures shouldn't do very well in facial recognition tests. So an experiment was designed: First, Williams kids were presented a picture of a face. Then they saw six other faces from a variety of angles, and in a variety of lighting conditions, from deep shadow to bright light. Only one of the six pictures was of the same person. Which one, the researchers asked, is it?

Williams kids performed just about as well as regular adults on the test, despite their profound difficulties with spatial skills. They had a "dramatic" ability to discriminate unfamiliar faces, Bellugi and her colleagues said. This suggested, once again, that some different system in the brain was responsible for the ability to perceive faces, something at least partially separate from the brain systems that governed other spatial skills. This excited Bellugi; this extremely unusual pattern of mental peaks and valleys spilled over into the spatial realm as well as the verbal one.

It's likely that face perception, and the ability to understand the emotional states of others, are closely tied to the ability to form and maintain social relationships, speculated Barbara Pober, a clinical geneticist at Yale University School of Medicine. Perhaps that had something to do with their friendliness and hypersociability.

Bellugi and her colleagues began doing tests to try to tease out the physical differences in Williams syndrome brains. They found that the Williams brain is only 80 percent as large as a regular brain; but they couldn't find any obvious differences in the cerebral cortex—the part responsible for higher functions—that might explain Williams's odd peaks and valleys of ability. The most striking difference they found was in the cerebellum, a part of the brain located at the base of the skull that controls coordination and muscle movement. Parts of the Williams cerebellum were significantly larger than the same areas in Down syndrome brains—and even larger than in regular brains. No one knew what it meant.

Bellugi and her colleagues published a chapter about Williams in a book in 1988, and her work would motivate a large group of behavioral researchers to devote themselves to studying Williams. Williams became a rallying ground for those who believed in the "modular organization" of intelligence—the idea that different mental abilities are independent and separable, much like the pieces of a sectional sofa. Together, they might make a stunning piece of furniture; but even if one or two are taken away, you still have something that works essentially like a sofa.

Didn't that seem to be the story of Gloria? Gloria, who couldn't make change for a dollar, but who could charm a *Los Angeles Times* reporter with girl talk. "Do you have a boyfriend? I do. And you know what? One day he was in my swimming pool and he splashed water on me. . . . Did you like the lipstick I had on yesterday? Did you think it was pretty? I like to put on makeup. . . . "

Gloria, who was not as loquacious as many Williams people, but who could still articulate an emotional truth with devastating accuracy. What she liked best about singing "Somewhere over the Rainbow" was, it made her feel less lonely. "The verse I love is, 'Where troubles melt like lemon drops, away above the chimney tops, that's where you'll find me. . . .'"

Gloria could answer the question "Are you happy with your life?" more honestly than most people he'd ever met: "Sometimes I'm not happy," she said. "Sometimes people tease me on the bus. Sometimes I want to do things other people can do that I can't do. But when I'm performing, I try not to let those things get to me too much, because then I won't be able to think of all the good things coming up."

Howard felt like he was beginning to understand his daughter in a much deeper way. Gloria, and this Williams syndrome, were indeed fascinating.

Gloria's miniconcerts became a big draw at Williams picnics and at Sally Meersman's Christmas parties. People called Gloria a savant, a miracle, a wonder, and Howard noticed that Gloria was far better at recalling everyone's names than he was.

Hungry for more information, Howard attended a few meetings. They were often held in dreary conference rooms and focused on the dire problems Williams children might face: narrowing of the aorta; narrowing of the renal artery, which supplies blood to the kidneys; systemic high blood pressure, which increases the risk of heart disease and stroke, and can lead to congestive heart failure, kidney disease, and blindness. Howard began referring to the doctors and researchers as "The Prophets of Doom." Everything was about what Williams children couldn't do, not what they could do. Simple concepts like "bigger" and "smaller" stumped Williams people, the researchers said; Howard believed this was often more a function of how the questions were asked than how they were answered. A researcher would soon show Gloria a picture and ask, "Which has the most wood?" Gloria would freeze, unable to answer. Howard later fetched a banana, cut it into two pieces—one bigger, one smaller—and asked Gloria which was bigger. Gloria understood this perfectly, grabbing the larger half of the banana and smiling mischievously. Williams people *could* understand concepts, Howard believed, if they were clearly explained and tied to something in their own experience.

Howard continued to attend the meetings, though, because he could usually convince the organizers to allow Gloria to sing during breaks. She was like a lightning bolt in the gloom, and her smile during the applause never failed to make any aggravation worth it.

Sally Meersman and her colleagues at the Williams Syndrome Association decided that Gloria simply *must* sing at the 1990 national conference in Boston. It would be marvelous if the Lenhoffs could do a session explaining how they managed to help Gloria reach her level of professionalism, Sally said. It would really lift the spirits of parents and children alike. Gloria would show everyone how much a Williams person could accomplish with hard work and dedication, and she could end the conference with fireworks by singing at the closing banquet.

The convention was going to be held at the Boston Park Plaza Hotel, one of the most grand and historic in New England. Gloria would have a receptive audience, and something to look forward to. They had many friends and relatives in the Boston area, and it would give them a chance to talk to other parents about how very much a handicapped person can accomplish.

Running right before the parents' meetings would be a professional symposium where educators, doctors, and scientists presented the latest research on Williams. Parents were excluded from these scientific gatherings, but if Howard was going all the way to Boston, he wanted in. So he wrote an abstract that he called "Musical Ability of a Williams Syndrome Adult: Case of One" and used his professional prerogative as a research biochemist and a professor at the University of California to gain access to the sessions and present it.

As the folks at the Williams Syndrome Association would soon learn, it was hard to say no to Howard Lenhoff.

{chapter 6}
AN EERIE APTITUDE

The Lenhoffs were transported back to the Old World. The hotel was all rosy brick and red awnings, and its cavernous lobby seemed to shimmer as if dipped in gold. It was near the Boston Commons and trendy shops and art galleries; a short walk to the theater district, the State House, Freedom Trail, and Beacon Hill. Their rooms were tidy in a European kind of way, and Gloria was thrilled to discover she'd have her very own bathroom, all to herself. It seemed spectacularly grand.

Things had come a very long way since the Williams Syndrome Association's first convention in 1984 in San Diego—a fly-by-the-seat-of-your-pants affair so tenuous they didn't even have enough money to pay rental fees to the hotel, and had to pass a hat through the crowd during the banquet. This time the Williams Syndrome Association had close to two thousand members, with ballrooms booked and hundreds attending.

The forbidden professional conference began a day before the regular convention, so the Lenhoffs were among the first Williams families to arrive. There would be presentations on genetics and endocrinology, nephrology and gastroenterology, behavior and neurology, as well as abstracts on calcium-regulating hormones, cognitive development, and platelet-derived growth factor. Howard toted Gloria's accordion into the conference room and took a seat in front with the other scientists, psychologists, and physicians, while Sylvia and Gloria took seats in back. Soon a Williams Syndrome Association board member insisted that Sylvia and Gloria leave; the policy was that no family members were allowed to attend the scientific meetings. They were meant for professionals, and professionals only. Sylvia explained that Howard *was* a professional and that she and Gloria were part of his presentation. There was a flurry of furrowed brows, and the association's outgoing president, Gordon Biescar, had to intervene and give them the OK to stay. Howard would get fifteen minutes to speak. Sylvia and Gloria moved up to the front row as he took the podium.

"Musical Ability of a Williams Syndrome Adult: A Case Study," Howard began. "Howard M. Lenhoff, Department of Developmental and Cell Biology, University of California, Irvine."

Howard joked that they were probably lucky that they had never heard of Williams syndrome when Gloria was growing up. If they had known all that she wasn't able to do, she might have never done all that she did.

Howard's paper barely covered half a sheet of paper, single-spaced.

"The subject, GML, was born premature in 1955 before the symptoms of Williams syndrome were defined. She suffered from 'colic' for nearly five years, was diagnosed soon after birth with a heart murmur, was tested as educably retarded at age seven. When she was twelve, her parents gave her an accordion, which she picked up and played immediately with no instruction or practice. At that time GML was also singing and retaining complex Hebrew melodies. After trying a number of voice and accordion instructors, a few were found who would teach a mentally retarded child who, to this day, cannot read music. Twenty years later, GML was recognized as having perfect pitch, has a repertoire of over one thousand musical pieces ranging from classical opera for soprano and musical theater pieces, to Beethoven's 'Moonlight Sonata' and modern rock on the accordion. GML, now an experienced professional TV and university performer and a Jewish cantor, will present two examples of her repertoire during the platform presentation of this report."

He invited Gloria to the podium. The scientists watched as she rose from her seat and walked as quickly as she could with her awkward gait. Howard helped her strap on the accordion and she jolted the somber crowd with the "Beer Barrel Polka," following up with the same song that concluded *Bravo, Gloria*, the short aria "Voi che sapete" from *Le Nozze di Figaro*.

The scientists politely applauded. How can Gloria hit all those high notes, one researcher asked, when one of the traits of Williams syndrome is a deeper voice? Twenty-four years of professional singing lessons and lots of practice, Howard answered.

A woman named Georgie Jacobus made her way to the podium. Georgie, an extraordinarily articulate woman with Williams syndrome who would soon serve as the Williams representative on the Williams Syndrome Association's board of directors, hugged Gloria and said, *"You* are *Bravo, Gloria!"*

Then she turned to the scientists with urgency in her voice. "I'm not used to microphones, but what I'm here to say is *wow*," Georgie said. "I am a very religious person and maybe a lot of people may not understand why, but my talking to you helps me understand what goes on in my own life, because inside I am a very angry person. A very emotional person. Because I get fed up with doctors who tell me that it's all emotional, and not physical.

"I put myself in a position last April to go into a place where I thought that they would help me. And all they did was to tell me that I was mentally retarded until the last week when I left. And that was when they found out that I had a thyroid condition. Can you imagine a person who has chronic pain being laughed at by a neurologist because he or she is in chronic pain? We are human beings just as much as anybody else.

"What chronic patients need is a lot of love and care, [to be] held close when they cry, and not have a doctor say, 'What is your complaint today, baby?' This is what I hear all the time with doctors. 'What is your complaint?' The problem is, we have problems, not complaints. We have a medical disorder that we need to fight. . . . These people who are out here this week need you more than you will ever know. . . .

"It hurts. It's painful . . . when you find out that you have Williams syndrome, and people laugh at you, and parents don't understand who you are. And Gloria, I want to tell you something. I am very proud of you for coming up here today and doing what you are doing.

"I saw a little child on the plane who is normal. I was able to hold her. Hold her in my arms. Rub her hair. And think, God, how I would love to have a child of my own. God, would I love to be loved by a man."

Georgie fought back tears.

"Excuse my anger. But I am frustrated. And I know you people are very tired of hearing all these things. But I love you all very much. And that's why I came. Because this is the best present anybody could get. To be able to talk to people who love you, and realize that you are just not mentally ill. Thank you very much."

Howard was deeply moved. Georgie was so insightful, so eloquent, so articulate. So fully human, in so much pain. In spite of Williams syndrome? Because of it? Her words would haunt most everyone in that room.

Colleen Morris was one of the scientists in that room. She had been working with Williams people for years, but she had never met one as eloquent as Georgie, or as musical as Gloria.

In her professional life, Morris was a pioneer. A new field

called "genetic counseling" was in its infancy in 1975 when she entered the master's program at Sarah Lawrence University—one of only a handful like it in the country. Morris would learn how to screen men and women who were considering having children for a variety of birth defects, genetic disorders, and inherited conditions. She would learn to identify couples at risk, analyze inheritance patterns and chances of recurrence, and explain it all to couples who might be getting terrible news. After two years as a genetic counselor, she discovered that the part she liked best was the puzzle. The diagnostic challenge. Birth defects fascinated her. What went wrong? How did they happen? Why did they occur at all?

That led her to medical school at Loyola University's Stritch School of Medicine in Chicago, a pediatrics residency in Phoenix, and a fellowship in genetics at the University of Utah. Morris had been seeing patients for only a short time when a child came in with the characteristic elfin face, health troubles, and social charms that characterize the disorder she had learned about in school—and Morris was quickly able to make a diagnosis of Williams syndrome. It was so early in her career and she was so excited she was able to spot it that she launched into a speech telling the child's mother everything she knew about Williams. The mother listened patiently, then asked one question: What happens when they grow up?

Morris looked at her blankly. She had no idea what happened when they grew up.

Well, *do* they grow up? the mother asked.

Morris said that most of the literature she was familiar with had been written about children, not adults. That seemed to be its own, grim answer. Morris promised to do more research.

The anguish in the mother's question haunted Morris as she hit the medical library. She could find only a handful of reports dealing with Williams syndrome in adults. Two of them were autopsy reports.

She told her mentor about the paucity of information about adults with Williams, and they decided it would make an excellent research project. She would answer that mother's question.

Morris set out in search of Williams grown-ups. The national Williams Syndrome Association was still in its infancy, so Morris was left to her wits. She visited sheltered workshops, residential homes for the disabled, state mental institutions, hospitals where she pored over cardiology records. In the end, she found forty-four people with Williams, seventeen of whom were adults. One was severely retarded and in a state institution, which turned out to be quite unusual for Williams adults. Most, she discovered, worked part-time doing simple jobs, and many lived at home with parents who had to care for them as they would children. They couldn't seem to learn the skills they needed to live on their own: how to safely cook food, how to clean up, how to do laundry, how to read a bus schedule.

Morris had read about their loquacious personalities — but it was one thing to read about, and something else entirely to experience. It wasn't so much their warmth and friendliness that struck Morris as their extreme empathy, something that went far beyond the earnest "Hi! How *are* you?" She'd watch as a Williams person zeroed in on the shadows passing over his parents' faces as they worried about the future, as they rushed to aid someone who had tripped and fallen, or to soothe someone who was crying. They were keenly attuned to the distress of others and wanted to offer comfort. She thought it uncanny, this genuine concern they had for the feelings of others. But she also saw adults with high levels of anxiety, people who were technically "mentally retarded" but quite aware enough to know that they were different, that they couldn't do the things everyone else could do, and they felt deeply frustrated by it.

Morris spent three years on the project and finished her research in 1986. The answer to that mother's plaintive question was published in the journal *Pediatrics*:

The natural history of Williams syndrome, including medical complications, growth patterns, and problems in adulthood, was investigated.

A growth pattern characterized by delay in the first four years of life, catch-up growth in childhood and low ultimate adult height was found.

Despite multiple medical problems in infancy, including feeding problems, failure to thrive, colic, . . . mean age at diagnosis was 6.4 years.

Developmental disabilities and cardiovascular disease were the major concerns in childhood. The older children developed progressive joint limitation and hypertonia [extreme tension of the muscles and arteries]. Adult patients were handicapped by their developmental disabilities. Hypertension, and gastrointestinal and genitourinary problems [relating to genital and urinary organs] occurred frequently.

Independent living and competitive employment were limited less by the individual's physical problems than by the psychologic and adaptive limitations. Williams syndrome is a progressive disorder with multisystem involvement.

The research was dispassionate. Morris's heart was not. She wanted to know why. What caused Williams syndrome? How did it happen? Her love of puzzles impelled her to find out.

At the professional conference in Boston, Howard and Sylvia listened as Morris said that she and her colleagues were zeroing in on the heart defect so often associated with Williams, supravalvular aortic stenosis (SVAS). This dangerous narrowing of the aorta was also seen in patients who had not a trace of Williams syndrome—and it passed through families, from parents to children. That told scientists that SVAS had a genetic component.

Morris teamed up with Mark Keating, a physician researcher at the University of Utah, and Greg Ensing, a cardiologist at Indiana University. The first thing they did was search for families that had SVAS running through the generations. They took blood samples. Did physical exams. Performed cardiology tests. And studied the data carefully, trying to find the common link. Their working hypothesis: there was some gene important to cardiovascular development that was involved in both SVAS and Williams syndrome. They expected there would be two different mutations involved, one that caused Williams syndrome and another that caused SVAS. They expected to have the answer soon.

As soon as the professional session ended, the parents' conference began. Howard, Sylvia, and Gloria entered the hotel lobby and discovered mounting pandemonium: the Williams families were arriving.

Howard had been to a few Williams gatherings before, so he thought he knew what to expect. But the scene in the Park Plaza Hotel was something else. Not just a dozen or two Williams families meeting and greeting, but hundreds. The thrilled screeching of Williams kids greeting one another like long-lost kin was deafening. Many had seen *Bravo, Gloria!* and, as Williams people never seem to forget a face, Gloria was received as if she was a rock star.

Anne Louise McGarrah was in shock. She, like Gloria, was an adult, diagnosed with Williams very recently. As she looked around, she began to cry.

"I never had seen anyone who looked like me until just coming to this convention," she told a writer for *Discover* magazine. "I was shocked! It was like—there's a person who looks like me! I look like them. This is quite amazing."

Journalist Robert Finn was taken aback as well. He had heard about Williams syndrome from a philosophy of science professor who spoke of their strange peaks and valleys of ability. Finn was intrigued. He pitched the story to *Discover* magazine, and soon found himself in Boston, surrounded by hundreds of Williams people with all their strengths and weaknesses. He found Anne especially fascinating.

"I love to read," Anne told him. "Biographies, fiction, novels, different articles in newspapers, articles in magazines, just about anything. I just read a book about a young girl—she was born in Scotland—and her family who lived on a farm. I love to read books because I can put myself in that book and be in there with her and watch her go through these experiences."

Finn noted that Anne had difficulty telling left from right, but could play piano and recorder and cherished classical music. "I love listening to music," she told him. "I like a little bit of Beethoven, but I specifically like Mozart and Chopin and Bach. I like the way they develop their music—it's very light, it's very airy, and it's very cheerful music. I find Beethoven depressing."

Williams syndrome turns topsy-turvy our notions of intelligence, Finn wrote. "It is this strange mix of mental peaks and valleys that has begun to fascinate psychologists and neurobiologists. When they understand Williams syndrome, they figure, they'll take a giant step toward understanding normal mental processes."

The sessions were held in rooms named after Emerson, Longfellow, and Thoreau. They dealt with education, job opportunities, behavior management, IQ tests, how to be an empowered parent. Howard's heart went out to the many thin-lipped and overwhelmed parents who dutifully scribbled notes and collected articles. He remembered how he felt when Gloria was younger and they couldn't fathom her future; certainly, she achieved more than he expected in his wildest dreams. He wanted to grab all the parents and tell them: Don't dwell on what your child can't do! Raise your expectations! Find out what your child does well and run with it! Your child will surprise you. Gloria was living proof of that. He hoped that, when everyone heard her sing, she would teach that lesson more powerfully than lectures ever could.

Gloria always looked forward to performing, but this performance was something special. She slipped into a new outfit bought specially for the occasion: a bright pink skirt with matching pink jacket over a fancy white blouse. She carefully applied her makeup so her eyes were wide and dramatic and her lips a deep crimson, then she ran through her vocal warm-ups. In addition to the hundreds conference attendees, the Lenhoffs had invited dozens of aunts, uncles, cousins, and friends who lived near Boston, including an old high school buddy of Howard's, Bob Bashevkin, who sold food wholesale. Howard was hoping some scientists stuck around so they could hear Gloria sing more challenging and moving pieces than she did during their fifteen-minute presentation.

Howard dragged Gloria's twenty-six-pound accordion through the lobby, up the stairs, and into the hotel ballroom. The ceiling soared, dripping crystal chandeliers. Tables elegantly draped in white linen and appointed with gleaming silver filled the room. People smiled as Gloria wended her way to her table, and she waited as Williams Syndrome Association president Gordon Biescar welcomed everyone, then invited Gloria to the stage.

Howard had developed a strategy for these things: start light and fun, then wallop them with the heavy stuff so they can't forget. He helped Gloria strap on her accordion. She launched into a medley of lively Italian songs that turned into "Hava Nagila," then did an excerpt from Beethoven's "Moonlight Sonata" ("What would Beethoven say if he were here?" Howard cracked), then urged the children to sing along to "My Bonnie Lies Over the Ocean," "When the Saints Go Marching In," and "You Are My Sunshine." Parents and children sang and clapped together, and Howard's face hurt from smiling. When he invited everyone up to dance, kids poured from their seats and gleefully obliged.

Then it was time for the big guns. Gloria put away her accordion and left the stage. Howard introduced a pianist from the New England Conservatory of Music, who took the bench before a luminous black grand piano. Gloria returned and took her place beside the piano, clasped her hands together, tucked her chin in the way Barbara Hasty had taught her, and sang the first crystalline notes of Mozart's "Voi che sapete." Then Schubert's art song "Heidenroslein," in German; "Musetta's Waltz," from Puccini's *La Bohème*; and "Somewhere over the Rainbow." As an encore, she sang Schubert's "Ave Maria," and was received with a standing ovation.

Some people rushed up to shake Gloria's hand and tell Howard how much their children loved music, too. Others wiped tears from their eyes. A few said that, technically, Gloria's voice might not be perfect, but she could certainly do incredible things, given her limitations. Most of the scientists, Howard noted, were long gone. It was their loss, he told himself.

As Gloria was bowing deeply, that incredible smile on her face, Georgie Jacobus made her way to the front of the ballroom with a bouquet of colorful flowers. Georgie, the woman who scolded the doctors with her heartfelt speech, presented the blooms to Gloria and said, "We are lucky to have Gloria here. Gloria, you are *Bravo, Gloria* and I'm quite proud of you."

So was Howard. He took the opportunity to remind everyone that the next day, he, Sylvia, and Gloria would be happy to answer questions at the session on how to teach music to children with Williams syndrome. He hoped they would come.

Howard, Sylvia, and Gloria sat in the front row of the Arlington Room, waiting for the music session to begin. There were enough chairs for sixty or seventy people; they hoped that at least a couple of dozen would show up so it wouldn't look too deserted.

Soon, the chairs in the back of the room filled up. That forced people to sit in the front. Soon those chairs were gone, too. When the doors finally closed, some one hundred people were there.

Howard wasn't exactly nervous. Making presentations in front of crowds was the bread and butter of his career. But he was certainly surprised. When he made scientific presentations, he always had notes and slides illustrating his points. For this, though, he hadn't made such preparations. He thought they were just going to answer questions.

The moderator introduced the Lenhoffs, and Howard took the podium. He thanked everyone for inviting his family to the conference, and said he was pleased to have heard from so many parents that their children loved music as much as Gloria did. There was much room for exploration in this area, he said.

The barrage of questions began. *How did you first notice that Gloria had extraordinary abilities? What kind of instruments did you try? How did she learn? How did you find a teacher who wouldn't demand that she learn traditionally? Where were lessons held? Why the accordion, why not the piano? How long does she practice? Can she read music?*

Howard invited Sylvia to the podium; she was the expert on Gloria's early years. The first thing they noticed was Gloria's great attention span for music, even when she couldn't concentrate well on anything else, Sylvia said. A murmur of recognition rang through the audience. She explained how they showered Gloria with musical toys and rhythm instruments to encourage her, about how difficult it was to find music teachers. The accordion because, well, the piano seemed so big, and Sylvia didn't know anything about the accordion and thought it would be easy to play. No, Gloria doesn't read music. Sylvia felt that her daughter's ability to hear was so fast and acute that reading music would probably just slow her down and interfere with the process. And Gloria learned by listening, listening, listening.

Did music help improve her math? Sylvia almost chuckled. Er, no, she didn't believe so.

Did her sensitive hearing have anything to do with her abilities? Sylvia didn't really know, except that Gloria could usually tell who was singing an aria after hearing just a few phrases.

Was Gloria a savant? No, I don't think so, Sylvia said. I think she has an ability, a proclivity, that had to be developed. It took a great deal of time and hard work for Gloria to become the musician she is today.

Howard asked if other parents had noticed any exceptional hearing or musical ability in their children, and stories erupted like steam from a pressure cooker. Nearly every parent had a story about his child's ultrasensitive hearing. How it was impossible to whisper without them understanding every word, how they were deathly afraid of thunderstorms, how they hated balloons because the sound of them bursting was agony. Some kids could actually tell one car from another by simply listening to the sound of its engine: *That's a Toyota Corolla, Ma. That's a Honda Accord*. Others had similar skills with vacuum cleaners and lawn mowers. Howard would soon hear how Amanda Miller ran outside to see a plane flying overhead long before her mother could hear a sound, how she'd be in bed with her eyes closed and hear a helicopter and say, "Mom, that's a Bell 412" or "That's a Huey," and how she could tell which chopper belonged to which TV station. Amanda had a similar gift for freight train whistles; she knew the Amtrak from the Southern Pacific.

Many of the kids began picking out melodies on the piano, or making up songs, or beating out complex rhythms, at only two or three or four years of age. Sally Meersman's daughter, Mary, was so hypnotized by beautiful melodies that she would weep and whine. Ben, four, used music therapy to learn to walk, mother Terry Monkaba said. They played martial music until Ben couldn't help but jump up and march around in time with it. He was constantly banging on things with straws and pencils and could keep a remarkably steady beat.

Parents far from Boston and the Arlington Room were discovering the same thing. Sharon Libera's son, John, didn't speak until he was almost three—when he sang "Baa, Baa, Black Sheep." The startled Sharon saw that he loved music and arranged for piano lessons for him, and John was doing quite well.

Lori Sweazy of Minnesota had an astonishing experience when her son, Alec, was not yet three months old. She was playing a slow jazz song on the piano as Alec listened intently.

When she hit a whole note in the piece, Alec echoed the tone, perfectly on pitch, with a long, clear "ooooh." Strange, she thought.
She played the piece again. Again, he sang the note, perfectly on
pitch. His eyes fixed on hers. He smiled and wildly kicked his
legs. Lori felt as if he was trying to tell her something. Then she
took the chord down a step, just to see what he would do. He
matched that note, too. "I just got chills," she said.

Mom Kristine Hendryx had a similar experience. She'd sing
to baby Mary when Mary was still in the crib—random notes,
nothing familiar. Mary would not just sing the notes back—perfectly on pitch—but she'd actually finish the tunes. Like she was
composing or something. Mary was only three.

Jason Dennis, twenty, was already a drummer so good that
he played in rock 'n' roll bands around town in Mississauga,
Ontario. Tests would soon place him in the top echelon of those
with drumming ability.

Howard was trying to make what he considered a very important point in the Arlington Room that day: discover your child's
interests and abilities, hone in on them, and help them grow. But
someone mentioned his child's love for athletics, and the discussion veered off into a detailed account of soccer games and cheer-
leading and the difficulty of getting fair and equal access on the
playing field.

Howard bit his tongue. He felt that they had missed his point.
Williams kids might have fun playing sports, but he had never
met one who could seriously compete with regular athletes. It
wasn't like that with music. Gloria could seriously compete on the
playing field of music. She had abilities that regular musicians
wished they had.

He tried to steer the conversation back to music, inviting
Gloria to the podium. *How do you learn? What advice do you have for
others?* The questions were too complicated for her, and she had a
difficult time answering. It pained Howard to watch her, because
she wanted so dearly not to disappoint. He quickly asked her to

play and Gloria rushed with great relief to her accordion, answering the only way she really knew how: in song. She played "When You're Smiling" (the whole world smiles with you), and ended with a French musette called "Jose," often played in cabarets. What more, really, was there to say?

One of the organizers of the convention was a striking woman named Kay Bernon. While others were harried and hassled with convention chaos, Kay exuded an otherworldly poise and calm. She was married to Peter Bernon, heir to a dairy fortune; they wintered in Wellesley, summered in Nantucket, and regularly appeared in the Boston society columns. Peter Bernon was known for being keen on Bentleys, and the family was on the front lines of philanthropy. Peter Bernon's grandfather started a dairy in 1931 that grew into an industry force and earned a reputation as an ideal corporate citizen. Bernon and his brother, Alan, were the ones locals turned to for help when students needed help paying for college, when the town common needed renovation, when the annual Fourth of July parade needed a boost. The Bernons felt that when a business was successful, it was an obligation and a privilege to give back.

In 1983 Kay and Peter's second son, Charles, was born. They soon became concerned that he wasn't developing normally, and when Charles was a year old, geneticists made the diagnosis of Williams syndrome. The Bernons had the means to give Charles the best of everything, but found they still had to fight to keep him in classes with regular kids, still had to help him negotiate the delicate social interactions of children, still had to battle the crushing evil of low expectations. Kay was scolded by a teacher for trying to explain to Charles about the conflict in the Middle East; the teacher felt that the details of war and religion were far beyond him. It enraged her.

This convention, and meeting Gloria, changed how she saw the future for Charles. All Gloria had achieved, despite her disabilities, gave Kay hope. If Gloria could do so well, perhaps Charles could do well, too. The Lenhoffs packed up and left Boston, feeling they had done their job.

But for all the accolades, the Lenhoffs also left behind seeds of discontent. Gloria was inspiring, a few parents whispered, but she was obviously the exception, not the rule. She was a savant. It was ludicrous to think that other Williams people could be like Gloria.

♪   ♪   ♪

It seemed there was a star on Howard's shoulder, and 1991 was shaping up to be a memorable year. After more than fifteen years of lobbying the government of Israel to give refuge to the oppressed and nearly destitute Ethiopian Jews, all those endless phone calls, meetings, letter-writing campaigns, and media interviews had finally paid off. Israel had airlifted some fourteen thousand people from Addis Ababa and taken them to Israel, their new home. Howard was ecstatic.

But the euphoria was not to last long. Shortly afterward, Gloria was on her way to work, changing buses to get from Costa Mesa to the preschool in Yorba Linda. At 8:30 AM, the phone rang in the Lenhoffs' home. Howard answered. Is this the Lenhoff family, parents of Gloria Lenhoff? a stranger asked. An icy dread rose in Howard: he summoned Sylvia to the phone, sensing this was the call all parents dreaded.

Gloria's inability to calculate velocity and distance collided tragically with an inattentive driver while she was crossing the street. She was hit by a car and dragged fifty feet. Her hip was shattered. So was her wrist. She was gashed and bruised and bloodied, and in the UCI Medical Center's emergency room.

Howard and Sylvia found her lying in a bed in the hallway awaiting x-rays and MRIs. Only her black-and-blue face was visible above the sheets. She was in pain, and frightened, but relief spread over her face when she saw them. Howard and Sylvia were ushered to an office where they could make phone calls, cancel their airline tickets to Minnesota, where Gloria was to perform for a Williams Syndrome Association regional convention, and have some privacy. Howard chalked up the VIP treatment to an error in the UCI phone directory: he was listed as "vice chancellor for student affairs," when he was actually "faculty assistant to the vice chancellor."

Gloria was in the hospital for three months, her health fragile, her parents sometimes fearing she wouldn't pull through. They stood sentinel in her room twenty-four hours a day: Sylvia by day, Howard by night. A friend sent a seven-member gospel group to her room to lift their spirits; Bernie played guitar and sang as she harmonized; Howard's students visited, as well as friends, rabbis, ministers, and pastors, and soon the walls were covered with cards and posters, the shelves overflowing with stuffed animals and flowers. Most of Gloria's doctors had never had a Williams patient before and didn't know how to deal with one; Howard took to posting stories about the syndrome all around her bed, in English and Spanish, to help educate them. Howard was trying to teach his From Conception to Birth class the day surgeons were fusing Gloria's hip fragments together; the operation dragged on for eleven hours. Finally, the class projectionist broke in and announced on the loudspeaker that Gloria's operation was a success. Everyone applauded, and Howard left for the hospital. There were life-threatening blood clots and drug complications, and it took nearly a year for Gloria to fully recover from the accident. And the pain wasn't just physical; she had to cancel several performances that had been booked, and that just added to the hurt.

Gloria was in physical rehabilitation, using a wheelchair and crutches, when an elegant note card landed in the mailbox on Robin Hood Lane, bearing a stamp of Queen Elizabeth. It was from Lady Cynthia Cooper in England. A dozen years before,

Lady Cynthia's daughter, Claire, was diagnosed with Williams, and she and her husband began Britain's support group and information clearinghouse for parents of Williams children. Word of Gloria's inspiring performances had spread across the Atlantic, and Lady Cynthia hoped the Lenhoffs would be able to attend the Williams syndrome convention in Central England's Stoke-on-Trent later that year. Stoke-on-Trent was a charming town and England's epicenter for pottery and bone china production. The great names of British china were there—Wedgwood, Spode, Portmeirion, Aynsley—and it would be wonderful if they could attend.

The Lenhoffs weren't keen on making such a long trip while Gloria's health was still fragile, but Gloria was eager to sing again before the crowds. Howard had also developed a taste for good bone china from his boyhood days as a salesman in his parents' gift shop, and he looked forward to seeing "china country." The Lenhoffs accepted the invitation and made plans to travel early to visit friends in Oxford, where they had lived for a time when Howard was a senior research fellow at Jesus College. Gloria would play her accordion in the central square and raise hundreds of British pounds for MENCAP, England's national charity for the mentally handicapped.

Stoke-on-Trent was a maze of winding streets lined with red brick buildings, Tudor manses with pointy roofs and impeccably manicured gardens. The conference was at the Grand Hotel, a classically British endeavor with dark wood furniture, somber paintings, wainscoted walls, and chandeliers that cast a buttery glow. As the Lenhoffs settled down to dinner at the hotel restaurant, a young man named Jeremy Colborne spotted them from across the room and made a beeline for their table. Jeremy, eighteen, also had Williams syndrome. He was reedy, with a dash of black hair, and delightedly welcomed Gloria to England. He, too, would be performing at the final banquet. He played the electronic keyboard, and looked forward to hearing her sing.

Why wait? he suggested. Do get your accordion, and we can play now, he urged Gloria.

Howard sighed. When they finished their meal, he dragged Gloria's accordion into a lobby alcove, while Jeremy and his mother set up his keyboard. Jeremy launched into songs that Gloria had never heard; she listened intently, picked up the melodies, and began weaving in harmonies. People started to gather. Gloria then played some songs Jeremy had never heard, and he harmonized as well. It struck Howard as incredible that two people with such profound disabilities could have such a keen second sense about music. Within an hour, families jammed the makeshift jam session, their Williams syndrome children dancing with abandon. It might have gone on like that all night, but a manager appeared shortly before midnight and asked everyone to break it up.

The British conference was very much like the Boston conference, with presentations of the latest scientific research and parental sessions on how to be an effective advocate. Gloria, however, was living for the final banquet, which would be her first major public performance since her accident.

Joining Gloria and Jeremy on the bill was a boy named Andrew. Andrew didn't sing, but he had a large repertoire of classical and popular pieces that he played on the electronic organ. He struck Howard as remarkably precise, never missing a note. Howard smiled as Andrew's mother sneaked up behind him with a crib sheet of songs and suggested what he might play next; Howard so often did that with Gloria. It seemed that these Williams kids froze when asked in a general way to play something; they needed a specific title — "Somewhere over the Rainbow," "Hava Nagila" — or they became paralyzed by the sheer number of songs they knew, or an inability to choose one over the other.

Gloria improvised duets with Jeremy and Andrew, then soloed. "God Save the Queen" had long been in her repertoire as

"My Country 'Tis of Thee," but she had never performed it in England. She was flustered when everyone leapt to their feet as she began to sing; it was the national anthem, after all. She smiled with surprise as they all sang along. But it was when Jeremy launched into one of his original songs that something inside Howard seized. "Old Joe Stalin," Jeremy called the song. It was an irreverent satire on the newly disintegrated Soviet Union, a ragtime sort of tune that seemed utterly, impossibly advanced for someone who was mentally retarded. Howard's and Sylvia's eyes met. This was odd. Extremely odd. Gloria was a talented musician. But there were other Williams people with talents as great, maybe greater.

Howard and Sylvia had fitful rests that night. Something strange was going on. Gloria. All those kids at the Boston conference who sang before they could speak and picked out harmonies on the piano before they could walk. And now, Jeremy and "Old Joe Stalin." Could it all be coincidence?

Howard was a scientist. He had watched Gloria every day for nearly forty years, not for the two or four or six hours that most scientists observed their subjects. He knew that what he was seeing was real, and Sylvia agreed with him. They became convinced that, somehow, Williams syndrome and music were linked.

Some would consider it preposterous. Some might question their objectivity. They were, after all, talking about their own daughter. But it was there. They were certain of it. The trick would be gathering the evidence and convincing everybody else.

{*chapter 7*}
AND MUSIC FOR ALL

H oward hit the library with a newfound ferocity. He combed through articles and databases on Williams, seizing upon scant bits of information: A 1964 report on the psychological characteristics of Williams that noted, in passing, that each of the children were "musical." An account written in 1985, in which a child said music was his "truest love." A 1987 study saying that Williams children easily learn songs. Letters and articles in the Williams Syndrome Association's own newsletter, where parent after parent noted his or her child's great love for music. Right under his own nose, Bernie was helping Gloria make a recording of British music to send to the families who attended the conference in Stoke-on-Trent—everything from Purcell to the Beatles—titled, "To My U.K. Friends, With Love."

More recent studies confirmed what he had heard from parents at the Boston convention—that a "psychophysical feature" of Williams is an unusual sensitivity to sound. About 95 percent of Williams people had hyperacusis. That meant that sounds considered loud to regular people were painful to Williams folks, and/or that Williams folks could hear soft sounds that others couldn't perceive. It was as if the volume control on their ears was stuck on "high."

In his research, Howard came across paintings of pixies from the nineteenth century by James Doyle, uncle of Sir Arthur Conan Doyle of Sherlock Holmes fame, and was struck by how similar they looked to Williams people. He did more library sleuthing and learned that historians believe that folklore, to a great degree, is based on real-life situations. One historian suggested that the story of Hansel and Gretel may have originated in times of famine, when parents sacrificed children to improve their own chances of survival. Howard stumbled upon a work called "Facial Folklore," asserting that in European folklore, fairies, elves, or other subhuman beings would steal healthy human children and leave their own physically deformed or mentally retarded offspring in their stead. Howard began to wonder if ancient folktales featuring magical "little people" had a biological origin, and might have been modeled on people with Williams syndrome, long before anyone knew that Williams syndrome existed. That these sprites were often musicians who enchanted people with their melodies bolstered Howard's confidence. A colleague even theorized that the large, pointed ears so often seen on illustrations of fairies might represent the sensitivity to sound so often seen in Williams people. Britain had its fairies, elves, and sprites. Arab literature described *jinnis*. North American Indians had *pukwudgies*. Africans had *yumboes*. From one end of the globe to the other, these mystical beings shared a set of traits: They were small, kindhearted, and loved children. They were extremely sensitive; had a passion for music, song and dance; were fascinated by circles and spinning objects; were orderly; and worried about the future.

When Howard shared his theory with other Williams parents, some were offended. Pixies? Elves? Fairies? They found the analogy between their children and creatures of medieval fantasy to be insulting. Some in the Williams Syndrome Association began to conclude that Howard was reaching too far, and that he was, in fact, a little bit wild.

One thing was certain: the controversy over Howard's paper on the "Pixie Theory" sparked a lot of interest and got people talking. Gordon Biescar appreciated that. Gordon had the deep drawl and easygoing demeanor of a guy from the outskirts of Houston; his son, Alex, had been diagnosed with Williams when he was six months old. Gordon was leaving his post as president of the Williams Syndrome Association, but was going to ramp up the work of the separate Williams Syndrome Foundation. While the association was primarily a support service for parents, the foundation would dedicate itself to funding scientific research and doing long-term planning. It had only four thousand dollars in the bank, but it had big plans for the future. This made many in the association nervous, worrying that the two organizations would trip over each other competing for scarce time, money, and resources. Biescar invited Howard to join the foundation's board of directors. Howard accepted, and within a year was elected president.

That's when University of Nevada researcher Colleen Morris called, appealing for money. Howard had met her at the Boston convention, she reminded him. Morris and her colleagues were closing in on the genetic underpinnings of Williams, and she needed five thousand dollars to pay part of an assistant's salary. She had already asked the Williams Syndrome Association, and had been directed to the foundation.

Howard knew the foundation didn't have that much money, but he also knew that universities were champions of the matching grant and would give a dollar if they could get a dollar. We'll give you $2,500, Howard told her, if you can get your dean to match it. She did. The grant was made.

It marked the beginning of infighting between the foundation and the association over purpose, vision, and how best to help those with Williams syndrome. Howard, as head of the foundation, was becoming a lightning rod for resentment.

♪　♪　♪

Sharon Libera was, by nature, a skeptic. She had a PhD in English literature from Harvard University, spoke her mind with soft precision, and was not one to suffer fools lightly. Sharon also had a sharp eye for detecting patterns, which would soon come in handy.

Her son, John, was diagnosed with a heart murmur when he was seven days old. But there was more amiss: John wouldn't look his parents in the eye. His head seemed to constantly turn to the left. The right side of his mouth drooped, and he wouldn't smile—until a worried Sharon took him to a pediatric neurologist to ask about it. John broke into a grin on the way out of the waiting room, putting the joke on her.

When John was nearly three and still not talking, Sharon and her husband took him to Boston for an exhausting and extensive evaluation. It took three days of poking, prodding, and testing. They were in their motel room on the last day—just before the nail-biting meeting at which the professionals would make their diagnoses—and John was zooming about in a hyperactive frenzy, grabbing everything he could get his hands on, causing Sharon to worry aloud that he would break something or hurt himself.

Shush, her husband told her. Shush and listen to him.

As John raced around, he was softly singing. "*Baa baa black sheep, have you any wool / Yes sir, yes sir, three bags full. . . .*" He sang it all the way through. From beginning to end. Lyrics intact.

Sharon was incredulous. How could a child possibly sing before he spoke?

The doctors said John had Williams syndrome.

Sharon was devastated. She was still wrestling through the pain months later when the family attended a harvest festival. A troupe of clog dancers thundered in percussive time on stage, keeping the fiddler's tricky rhythms with their heels on the downbeat. All Sharon wanted was for John to fit in, to be like regular kids, so when he rushed the stage and stomped alongside the dancers, Sharon was mortified. Her first instinct was to drag him back to his seat and reprimand him, until she saw, to her utter astonishment, that he could actually *do* it. He stomped his heels in time, keeping the beat right alongside the professional dancers.

My goodness, she thought. I don't think I could do that.

John obviously had a deep attraction to music and rhythm. His body tended to bop, even in perfect silence, as if keeping time to a song only he could hear. Sharon decided that, whatever else his education included, she'd try to encourage this propensity for music. From that day on, she bought him every musical toy she could find, much as Howard and Sylvia had done for Gloria so many years earlier. There were plastic trumpets, saxophones, and clarinets. There were harmonicas, drums, xylophones. There was a great din of tooting, bleeping, and blaring, and by the time John was five, he could play most any Christmas song you could name. He had trouble writing clearly and doing math, but he could dream up his own limericks: "Puppy, puppy, you ran so far / No matter, we'll find you wherever you are. / If you have a little scar, / Don't worry, we'll bring you into our car."

Sharon's mailbox was soon bulging with subscriptions to journals, pediatric magazines, and newsletters dealing with Williams. She wanted to know everything she possibly could about her son's condition. The folksy newsletter put out by the Williams Syndrome Association became a favorite for its in-the-trenches accounts and stray bits of advice from parents; Sharon's brow arched as she started to notice how often sentences like "Johnny loves to dance and sing" or "Suzie has a great passion for music" appeared in these first-person accounts, just as Howard's had. It was so common that she began reading the newsletter with pen in hand, circling each reference to music. Her collection of anecdotes grew large.

Then a case study in the journal *Compassionate Pediatrics* caught Sharon's eye. It was written by a parent struggling to do right by her Williams child, detailing the innumerable hours she spent driving her child to specialized doctors, specialized therapies, and specialized training. It mentioned, in passing, how far they had to go to find a piano teacher who taught by ear using the Suzuki method. The child was on book two and doing well, the article said.

Suzuki? Book two? Sharon had no idea what that meant, but she certainly understood playing music by ear. John was just in first grade, but he seemed to have a pretty good ear. Maybe this was something he could do. It seemed like a strange coincidence when she soon stumbled across an ad in the local newspaper for a lecture by a Suzuki method teacher. She went, with high hopes.

The teacher's name was Frigga Scott, and her talk included a piano recital by her youngest students, one of whom was blind. The music was delightful, the children loved being in the limelight, and Frigga Scott obviously knew how to work with handicapped children.

The Suzuki approach, Frigga explained, believes that children absorb music the same way they absorb language; slowly, almost automatically, one bit at a time. The "mother tongue" approach, they called it. It was developed by Dr. Shinichi Suzuki at his music school in Japan, and was a function of immersion, repetition, and intense parental involvement. Ideally, children began between ages three and six—the younger the better—and music was never, ever to be a chore. Lessons were full of fun and praise, no matter how small the child's accomplishments. It required an intense commitment from parents: they had to attend all the lessons alongside the child, take notes, practice with the child every single day, make sure the child listened to the pieces he was learning every single day.

Sharon rushed up after the presentation was over. She explained John's condition and asked if Frigga would consider teaching him. Frigga told her to bring John to her house for an audition.

An audition? Sharon was taken aback. John was only seven years old. He could play Christmas carols on his plastic saxophone . . . but an audition? Her stomach sank. Competitive and stressful situations weren't good for John. But something told her to take him anyway, and she stood by anxiously as Frigga asked him to sing "The Star-Spangled Banner." *The Star-Spangled Banner?* Sharon had never taught him "The Star-Spangled Banner." That song was nearly impossible to sing and everyone knew it—set as it was to the tune of an old English drinking song—and it was full of anachronistic language like "*What so proudly we hailed at the twilight's last gleaming.*" She held her breath, trying to prepare for disappointment, trying to figure out how she would comfort John afterward.

Then he opened his mouth and sang. "Oh say can you see by the dawn's early light / What so proudly we hailed at the twilight's last gleaming. . . ."

On pitch. In time. Sharon had no idea where he learned it. It must have been all those baseball games. He must have just absorbed it, as flowers absorb water, as the Suzuki people say.

Frigga was just testing John's ear, she explained lightly. John passed. Frigga would take him on as a student.

Sharon was delighted, throwing herself eagerly into creating a "musical home" for John, as the program required. She attended every lesson with him, took notes for him, made sure he listened to the pieces he was learning every single day, and became his at-home piano teacher, doing all his exercises by his side, even though she had never studied a musical instrument before. His little hands hovered over the keyboard, tentatively at first, then with greater and greater confidence: he progressed from "Twinkle, Twinkle, Little Star" to "Honey Bee" to minuets by Bach and Mozart. It was a tremendous investment of time and energy, but John loved it. He would become so completely absorbed in the music that nothing else seemed to exist. At first lessons were mercifully short, but as time went by they grew to forty-five minutes long, and John was absorbed the entire time.

Sitting in the anteroom of Frigga Scott's house at one of

John's lessons, Sharon noticed a pile of brochures about summer Suzuki institutes.

So that's what children who are seriously musical do in the summer, she thought. They go to camps where they train even harder and hone their skills. Wouldn't that be wonderful for John? That's exactly what he needs. Maybe she should send him.

But then reality pushed in: Socially, that sort of a setup would probably be very difficult for him. The kids might be competitive, or make fun of him, or reject him for being different. That would make him feel terrible.

As John played Frigga Scott's black grand piano, Sharon let herself get lost in a daydream. Wouldn't it be wonderful if there were a camp just for kids with Williams syndrome? No pressure, no competition, nothing that would frustrate them and make them feel like failures. Just fun. Wouldn't that be great?

John went on to take up the saxophone and joined the school band. He begged to join a junior drum and bugle corps, where he learned to play the horn and march to complex choreography at the same time. The bugle corps entered competitions and traveled all over the state. It surprised Sharon how much John could do if it involved music: his coordination, his self-confidence, even his math skills were better for it.

He was nearly twelve, and quite accomplished, when Sharon read a blurb in the Williams Syndrome Association newsletter, seeking parents who were interested developing music in their children. She bolted to attention. It was written by a man in California named Howard Lenhoff and included a phone number. Sharon called immediately and told Howard all about John; Howard told her all about Gloria; and they excitedly shared their independent observations and mutual conclusions. There *had* to be some sort of link between Williams syndrome and music, they agreed. How else to explain how people with such profound disabilities could excel in something as complex as music? They weren't prodigies, heaven knew. They had to work very hard. But when they did, they could achieve great things. They could *learn*. And once they learned, they never seemed to forget. Their love of music was so strong it had the power to transform their lives, to provide shape and meaning.

Sharon had never been very active in the Williams Syndrome Association. She was a big fan of the newsletter, but she lived in a small Massachusetts town and had never met another Williams family. Still, she felt very deeply that what she had learned about John and music could help other Williams families, and she wanted very much to share it with them. She had a crazy idea about filming John's music lessons so others could see for themselves and know how to proceed. She asked the Williams Syndrome Association for money to make a professional video; and, like scientist Colleen Morris, she was told to ask the foundation.

The powers-that-be at the association weren't too pleased that another parent was hopping on the musical bandwagon. They agreed that the kids loved music. But many felt that having an *attraction* to music wasn't the same as having a *talent* for music. It was interesting, this young John Libera and his Suzuki piano lessons. Certainly some children could benefit from it. But they just didn't believe that there were a lot of savants hiding in the Williams ranks. There just weren't a lot of Glorias and Johns out there.

The acrimony between the foundation and association left some nerves raw. The association started fielding phone calls from parents who were upset that their children didn't show any musical tendencies. *Another* thing wrong with them. It seemed cruel to let parents hope that their children could ever do what Gloria and John did. It would just lead to more heartache, and honestly, didn't they have enough? How many would rush out and arrange piano lessons for their kids, dreaming of little Mozarts, only to be crushed when the kids couldn't even learn to play "Chopsticks"?

Howard ignored the sniping and stayed tenaciously on message. He thought Sharon's video was a fine idea, and the Williams Syndrome Foundation kicked in one hundred dollars toward its production. *For the Love of Music* was shot mostly in Frigga Scott's living room, with John at her black grand piano. He stared at the keyboard through aviator glasses, playing a lilting Mozart minuet; Frigga showed him where to put his fingers, how hard to strike the keys, and at what tempo. He copied her perfectly.

"Do you know what this line means?" Frigga asked, pointing to the musical score.

"Ummmmmm . . . ," John responded, not wanting to disappoint her by saying no.

"If you're not sure, I'll tell you," Frigga said.

"OK," John said quickly.

"It means you get to use the damper pedal."

"Cool!" John replied, instantly doing as told. Dozens of copies of the video were made, and Sharon and Howard were gratified when a few people ordered them.

It was a start. A regional conference of the Williams Syndrome Association was to be held in Boston that year, and Howard asked the regional director for a few minutes on the program to discuss music and education. He was given the OK— until officials at the national association heard about it and his presentation was suddenly canceled. Angry, and even more determined, Howard decided to attend the conference anyway, to meet with Sharon and other parents interested in music, and to figure out how to better promote music in the Williams community. He and Sharon shared the same convictions: Music could be a path to a better life for Williams people, people who could do so much more than anyone expected. Others could achieve just as much as Gloria and John had, if they only got the chance. They had to provide that chance.

Before the conference, Howard met Sharon and John face-to-face. He joined them for a piano lesson at Frigga Scott's house, and was impressed with John's talent. He and Sharon discussed strategy, and headed with great purpose to the Boston meeting. Howard raised questions about music at most every session he attended. He talked about music to families in the lobbies and between sessions. He encouraged people to attend a meeting about music after the conference was over—a barbecue at the home of Milena Kalinovska, director of Boston's Institute of Contemporary Arts and mother of a Williams child—to brainstorm on how to bring music center stage for Williams families.

Resentment against Howard was building. He was overzealous, some parents said. He led Gloria around like a trained monkey, forcing her to perform. Who was this really about, her or him? Without his constant, overbearing attention, without him telling her which song to sing and when, she wouldn't be able to do anything. It was more about Howard, they whispered, than anything else.

The brainstorming session was sparsely attended. Kay Bernon, who was so impressed by Gloria's performance at the Boston convention, said she was interested, but couldn't make the meeting. Several others had conflicts. In the end, Howard, Sharon, and the Kalinovskas huddled among themselves. Sharon still had the vision that came to her that day in Frigga Scott's house, of a summer camp where John could go with people who were like him and play music for the sheer joy of it, developing his talents without pressure or competition. Howard's main interest was still a residential community where gifted handicapped people could get formal musical training, maybe even a degree, which had been his dream since Gloria's Hi Hopes years. He hoped that his university, UCI, would provide land if the Williams Syndrome Foundation could raise money for a building.

But those were mighty ambitious goals for the short-term. They should probably start more modestly, doing one-day workshops at the Children's Museum or the like. It was all brand new to them and they weren't really sure where to begin, so they agreed to spend the next year gathering information, focusing on a summer camp, and figuring out the next logical steps. They'd have to put everything together themselves, they were sure—location, staffing, program, logistics—and that would take time. It was an overwhelming, and exciting, prospect.

Howard said his good-byes to Sharon, John, and the Kalinovskas that Sunday afternoon and headed back to nearby Pittsfield, Massachusetts, to visit his mother. He had arranged to have breakfast the next day with his high school buddy Bob Bashevkin. Bob had been there when Gloria sang at the 1990 Williams convention in Boston, and he had a tender place in his heart for Gloria. Howard and Bob had played basketball in their youth—neither was terribly good—and Bob stayed on in tiny Adams, building up a successful wholesale food business. Bob sold bulk flour, beans, bread, and meat to colleges, jails, schools—anyone who needed a lot of it. Howard and Bob met at the local coffee shop in Adams—where Howard's niece was a waitress—to catch up before Howard flew back to California.

What's new with Williams syndrome? was one of the first questions Bob asked. Howard told him all about the meeting at the Kalinovska home and how they were going to spend the next year figuring out how to start a music camp for Williams people.

Really? Bob said. One of his wholesale food clients was actually a fancy arts camp nearby called Belvoir Terrace.

Belvoir Terrace was an exclusive and expensive endeavor on forty acres in historic Lenox, where literary legend Edith Wharton once lived. It catered to the daughters of the Park Avenue set, people who could spend six thousand dollars on seven weeks each summer. Belvoir recruited musicians from Juilliard, directors from Broadway, and prima ballerinas from the New York City Ballet to teach these privileged young women. Cellist Yo-Yo Ma, violinist Marylou Speaker, pianist Leon Fleisher, and conductor Benjamin Zander had all taught master classes there.

It was a proudly matriarchal enterprise. Belvoir began in the 1950s, after one of Edna Schwartz's daughters decided she wanted to be a ballet dancer. Edna searched for a place to send the girl over summer recess so she could hone her craft, but all Edna could find were camps featuring swimming, sports, and crafts. None offered serious training in the arts.

There must be other children like mine, Edna told herself. If she couldn't find an arts camp for her daughter, well, she'd simply start one.

Edna opened Belvoir Terrace in 1954, a time when few women dared run businesses of their own. She painted everything with varying shades of her favorite color—purple—and planted the grounds with purple flowers. Belvoir would enroll only girls. Edna wanted to open their eyes to wonder, to teach them to cherish beauty, to help them experience the preciousness of friendship. There would be intensive classes in art, dance, music, theater, tennis, swimming, and riding, and only the most motivated need apply. People thought Edna was crazy.

That, Howard thought, was his kind of person. Do you have a number where I can reach her? he asked as he headed to the Albany airport.

Howard called Nancy Goldberg, one of Edna's now-grown daughters, from a pay phone at the airport, dropping his friend's name.

Ah, she said. Bob. The guy who sells me meat.

We have an idea for a very unusual music camp, Howard said as the airport's public address system blared in the background. He explained about Gloria and John and the strange musicality of the others until the final boarding call for his flight trumpeted through the terminal.

Once you hear Gloria sing, you'll be impressed, Howard assured her.

Nancy was often asked to listen to someone's daughter sing or watch them dance or hear them recite Shakespeare. She knew that every parent thinks his or her kid is fabulously talented; and she knew not to dismiss them out-of-hand. Sometimes, experience had taught her, the parents were exactly right. She told Howard to call again when he got back to California and had time to talk.

Howard called again within days.

I am a scientist, he told Nancy. My daughter has an uncanny gift for music, and I have met other Williams people with that gift, too. Many of their parents don't know it, or won't see it, but I am certain it's there.

It seemed a natural next step in Belvoir's evolution: Belvoir had given women opportunities to grow and excel in the arts when such opportunities had been denied to them for centuries. Today, Williams people were in much the same straits as women had been half a century ago. Their potential was overlooked. Their talents were wasted.

He's pushy, this man, Nancy thought. I like him. She had never heard of Williams syndrome, wasn't sure that people with IQs of fifty could get much out of formal music training, and didn't know where she would find the time to host them even if she was inclined to do so. Her regular camp ran from June to August and was such a time-consuming endeavor that doing any more seemed quite overwhelming. Her instructors were working artists and athletes and musicians and dancers, not special education teachers. And Belvoir had never hosted a male camper before, much less a mentally disabled one. But Howard was so very passionate.

Howard urged Nancy to see for herself. There was a talented Williams boy who lived in Massachusetts, not too far from Belvoir, he told her. His name was John Libera, and he had been playing piano since he was seven. John and his mother, Sharon, could visit.

I look forward to it, Nancy said.

Sharon was excited and nervous as they drove through Lenox's quaint brick-and-clapboard downtown and turned onto Cliffwood Street. It was beautiful, lined with enormous houses and towering trees that must have been old during the Revolutionary War. Then, she saw it, perched high on an expansive lawn like some lordly castle: Belvoir Terrace.

It was an enormous, gothic mansion, with imposing turrets, spiky spires, and a steep, sloping roof. It was built in the 1890s for industrialist Morris K. Jesup, the man who became a millionaire in the railroad banking business and helped found the American Museum of Natural History. It was like no camp Sharon had ever seen, but rather a setting for some elegant period drama where a lady might idle time in a fancy parlor set with sterling silver and bone china.

Sharon found no such lady. Instead, she found Nancy Goldberg, a brusque, businesslike, no-nonsense woman in jeans and a T-shirt who didn't fuss over her short-cropped hair. Nancy had worked beside her mother, Edna, every summer since Belvoir opened in 1954—as swimming teacher, counselor, and now, as Edna was slowing down, as Belvoir's director. It was hard to believe it had been almost forty years. The place now boasted four dance studios, five theaters, ten art studios, twenty-four music studios, two pools, six tennis courts, and forty grand pianos, two of which were actually in bathrooms. It was a quirky place, Belvoir. Nancy's own daughter, Diane, had attended every year for her entire girlhood, and would go on to earn a master's degree in piano performance from Juilliard, a doctorate from the City University of New York, and to help run Belvoir with Nancy and her grandmother Edna. Belvoir was a dynasty.

First things first, Nancy said. Let's hear John play.

Sharon and John were led past two Moorish arches into the mansion's grand room, where floor-to-ceiling windows framed the lush green hills and flooded the place with light. A grand piano beckoned, and John took a seat on the bench.

His face seemed blank as he launched into Mozart's formal, floral Minuet in G, but his focus was entirely on the keyboard. The piece had a jaunty air and showy trills, and in the mansion's great room, you could practically see the glow of oil lamps and the blur of ladies twirling with stiff-collared gentlemen. John looked up, expressionless, when he finished. Nancy nodded. She was impressed, but didn't let on.

He's very well trained, she said. But he could use a little work on his technique.

Nancy wanted to see more. Camp was in session, she said. Would John like to visit some classes and play with the instruments? John's eyes lit up.

Nancy had been working with talented children for so long she felt she could spot them blindfolded. To them, music or art or dance wasn't just pretty or fun or something to do; it was like a true love, an object of intense desire, and the afflicted seemed to quiver when it was in close proximity, buzzing and snapping like live wires. That's what Nancy saw in John as he rushed about campus. He raided the woodwinds and the strings, charged the drums in the percussion room, stopped dead in his tracks at the sublime sound of aspiring opera singers warbling arias. He listened so intently that he seemed to ache with the very beauty of the music. It was uncanny, the way he responded, Nancy thought to herself. After so many decades tending to aspiring artists, she had never seen anything quite like it. She started introducing John around campus as a good pianist who might be coming to a special camp at Belvoir next year.

When Nancy spoke to Howard, she said she was impressed. But surely they couldn't all be like John.

Not now, Howard said. But with work, they could be.

Sharon soon returned to Belvoir with a larger group of Williams parents. If an environment can be healing, one parent said, this would be it. It would let us see what the kids are capable of and help us make plans for the future. It will also help the children realize they are capable of something. The parents loved Belvoir, and were eager to start.

Nancy was inclined to do the camp, but she worried. What about discipline? How would her staff manage these kids, take care of them? How much help did they need with the basics — washing, dressing, and feeding themselves? Howard and Sharon assured her that Williams kids were perfectly able to feed and dress themselves. They were also remarkably obliging, very eager to please, and happy to do as they were told. A potential problem, though, was getting from point A to point B on Belvoir's sprawling campus; Williams kids find it difficult to follow directions, so going from the percussion room to the piano room to the dining hall could cause confusion and tears. The steep hills would make it difficult for them to walk anywhere. Perhaps they could have counselors or teachers accompany them from place to place? Williams people also had a tendency to be anxious. Many had never been away from home for any length of time before. Parental supervision was probably a must for the youngest of them, and a good idea for others.

Howard, Sylvia, and Gloria soon flew to Massachusetts to visit Howard's mother. The next morning, they headed to Belvoir to meet Nancy. Instead of the mansion's great room, they wound up in the cluttered gatehouse, once the nerve center overseeing all who came and went to the estate. Now it was a tiny office stuffed with books, papers, and file cabinets. Nancy looked closely at Gloria: She saw a quiet woman with a faraway look, someone who didn't seem to be paying much attention to what was going on around her. Her reserve was a marked contrast to some of the others' exuberance.

Howard asked Gloria to stand up and sing a song for Nancy. Gloria clambered to her feet, took a deep breath, and launched into Puccini's "Musetta's Waltz," from *La Bohème*. Her voice exploded into the tiny space, and Nancy reacted physically, her body moving back a bit, as if she was being pushed. Gloria's diction in Italian sounded perfect; her emotional inflection, precise. Nancy listened to the vibrato; technically, it wasn't perfect— Gloria wobbled a bit—but she was still utterly remarkable. As Gloria sang on, Nancy's brow settled into a deep, incredulous furrow.

Gloria finished and took her bow. Howard locked eyes with Nancy.

Impressive, Nancy said. Let me hear another.

At Howard's prompting, Gloria sang "De vieni, non tardar," from Mozart's *Le Nozze di Figaro*. When she finished, Howard flashed her the smile of a proud father.

"I wouldn't have believed it if I hadn't seen it, that someone with an IQ of fifty-five could sing in Italian. It's crazy," Nancy would later say.

She was smitten. Guarantee me fifty campers at five hundred dollars a head, and I'll put together a weeklong program for next August, she told Howard.

Howard and Sharon were ecstatic. The vision they thought was years down the road was tantalizingly close to coming true. Giddy at their good luck, they promised Nancy they would find fifty campers for August 1994.

{chapter 8}

MAN ON A MISSION

When Howard returned to California, a message was waiting from Colleen Morris, the University of Nevada geneticist who said she was on the brink of unraveling the genetic underpinnings of Williams. Morris was the one who vowed to answer the questions, "What happens to Williams kids when they grow up? *Do* they grow up?" for the worried mother; she's the one who talked Howard and the Williams Syndrome Foundation into giving $2,500 to pay a lab assistant as they closed in on their target.

Now Morris and her colleagues had a big announcement to make, and she wanted the Lenhoffs to be in Las Vegas on August 30, so they could hear it. The philosophical and scientific implications of their findings were tremendous, and would launch scientists on an enormous new mission: trying to understand the links between gene, brain, and behavior. The questions raised were controversial. Uncomfortable. And fascinating.

Morris and her colleagues, Mark Keating at the University of Utah and Greg Ensing at Indiana University, had been playing genetic detectives, working backward from disease to gene. The disease was the dangerous narrowing of the aorta called SVAS that was so common in Williams people, but which was also found in people without a trace of Williams. The scientists had ferreted out families of normal intelligence where the disease ran through the generations, to evaluate alongside their Williams subjects. Other than the heart problems, the two groups were so different. What could be the common link?

The scientists took blood samples, did physical exams, performed cardiology tests, and carefully studied the data from both groups. Their working hypothesis: Some gene important to cardiovascular development was involved for both groups. They expected there would be two different mutations involved, one that caused Williams, and another that caused SVAS.

They were a little bit right, and a little bit wrong.

It made looking for a needle in a haystack look easy, as the genetic haystack was believed to be one hundred thousand genes strong at the time (though now it's known to be about thirty thousand). After years of scrutinizing chromosomes—time-consuming, painstaking, microscopic work—the researchers finally zeroed in on chromosome 7. Chromosome 7 held the key to Williams and SVAS alike.

Every cell contains twenty-three pairs of chromosomes, one set from the mother, one set from the father. These chromosomes contain DNA—the "blueprint of life"—and dictate everything from what color our hair and eyes are to how we manufacture red blood cells, digestive fluid, elastin, and so on.

Elastin is a vital protein. It's what enables tissue to expand and contract. Elastin is critical to healthy arteries, lungs, intestines, skin, and many other organs; and the gene for elastin is found on chromosome 7. Morris and her colleagues found that there was something very wrong with the elastin gene both for Williams people and for people of normal intelligence with SVAS.

For the folks of normal intelligence with the heart problems, a mutation was found in the elastin gene on one of the two copies of chromosome 7. That meant that, for every molecule of normal elastin they produced, they also produced one molecule of abnormal elastin. That led to a defective elastin protein, which led to rigid, inflexible tissue, which led to the dangerous narrowing of the aorta.

In a fascinating twist, things were different in Williams people. One elastin gene was fine. But the other was missing entirely. It was not mutated, as it was in the other group; it was simply gone. Deleted. Dropped. Cast aside like an old shoe. So Williams people didn't make as much elastin as the body needed to function normally. Suddenly the odd assortment of physical problems started to make sense. So *that* was why Williams people are so prone to heart problems, digestive problems, high blood pressure, early-wrinkling skin. The facial features. *That's* what happened when the body doesn't produce enough elastin. Morris and her colleagues talked about a practical impact this discovery would have for Williams families: an easy genetic test, which would lead to earlier diagnoses and more focused therapies for kids, so they could grow up to be their best.

Howard was obsessed with the simple matter of how the deletion happened. He had suffered with so much guilt for forty years, sure he and Sylvia were directly responsible for Gloria's problems. It was the early delivery, or the forceps, or the lack of oxygen during birth, as the doctors had said. Things that, if they had only been done another way, could have resulted in a startlingly different life for their daughter, and for themselves.

Morris's answer put an end to all that agonizing. Williams syndrome was a genetic hiccup. A mistake. An error. There was nothing parents could have done to cause it, and nothing they could have done to prevent it. The missing gene was probably dropped when the egg or sperm were made, and the deletion was there from the moment sperm and egg came together. It wasn't the parents' fault.

For the first time in forty years, something that resembled peace, and relief, filled Howard. *It wasn't our fault*, he thought.

Howard gathered his composure and told the press that the grant to Morris was the best investment the Williams Syndrome Foundation ever made, joking that the foundation had hit the jackpot in Las Vegas on just one try.

Soon Morris and her colleagues dropped their scientific bombshell: In Williams people, the genetic mystery went far deeper than just one gene missing from chromosome 7. Yes, one copy of the elastin gene was gone, *but so was a length of DNA on either side of it*. The deletion was about twenty genes long. They had no idea what those genes were for, or what they were supposed to do. They were genetic phantoms. Could they be at the root of the brain abnormalities in Williams people? Could they somehow be responsible for personality traits like friendliness, compassion, and sociability? Were they the source of their unique talents and bizarre intellectual profile—facility with language, inability to comprehend math? Was it true, as this was suggesting, that chemistry was truly destiny? Morris and her colleagues couldn't yet say, but they were afire with the questions.

The genetic detectives would now embark full bore on trying to trace the links between gene, brain, and behavior. Williams presented an unparalleled opportunity to probe the deepest mysteries of the human condition. It was, as one scientist would say, a geneticist's dream.

Howard felt wired. Infused with the kind of manic energy a person feels when the hidden pieces of a puzzle start to fall astonishingly into place. He was restless, impatient, eager to make something happen. He was certain that the deleted genes on chromosome 7 must have something to do not only with the strange personality quirks of Williams people, not only with their health problems and bizarre cognitive profile, but with their mysterious musical ability as well. He felt a compulsion; it must be studied. Scientists simply must branch into music.

He told Colleen Morris that he was sure that musical ability was somehow wound up with those missing genes. Why didn't some of her colleagues consider widening the scope of their inquiries?

Morris loved working with Williams people. It was one of the highlights of her life. By now she had spent more than a decade studying Williams patients, people of all different ages and ranges of ability, people from all over the country. Yes, several seemed musical—she could recall one child who played the piano by ear, another who dabbled with the guitar—but none had reached Gloria's level of accomplishment. Howard and Sylvia were a musical family. Howard played some guitar and, in his own estimation, could yodel pretty well. Sylvia played some piano. It made as much sense to suppose that Gloria inherited her musical ability from her parents as to think it was somehow tied to Williams syndrome. Talent, she felt, seemed no more prevalent in the Williams population than it did anywhere else.

Howard wished he could do the research himself, but he was a biochemist, not a behavioral scientist. He knew the hydra down to its last tentacle, but he was no authority on behavior and the brain. So he tracked down the psychologists, cognitive scientists, and researchers studying various aspects of Williams, trying to hook their interest. He urged them to quantify the anecdotal observations of musical ability reported by Williams parents and teachers; he even pulled together a list of those observations, published them in *Music Therapy Perspectives*, and distributed copies to the would-be researchers. "Whereas Williams children have short attention spans for most subjects, their attention span for listening to music and in participating in musical activities is long," it said. "Although most cannot read musical notation, some are said to have absolute and relative pitch. Some have an excellent sense of timing, as when two experienced vocalists were able to perform a complex classical duet nearly perfectly at their first practice. Some can retain long pieces of complex music in a variety of languages for years, even decades." He cornered scientists at professional meetings and conferences. Leading Williams researcher Ursula Bellugi had invited Gloria to her lab to sing for neurologist and author Oliver Sacks; she had seen the look on the Williams children's faces when Gloria played accordion; she knew what Howard was talking about. Bellugi agreed that music was an intriguing line of inquiry; but, unfortunately, she didn't feel it was her area of expertise. Most reactions from the other researchers were similar.

Howard found their lack of action frustrating and disturbing. He wanted scientists to quantify what he and Sylvia had seen, what so many others saw so clearly: that there was a link between Williams and music. If the researchers wouldn't open their minds, he would do an end run around them. He'd use all the lessons about political activism he learned while helping relocate the Ethiopian Jews and apply them here. He would become like an evangelist, attracting converts until the scientists could no longer ignore it. And how better to reach people in this era of mass communication than the mass media?

Howard launched a campaign to get newspaper and TV and radio people to pay attention to music and Williams syndrome. If they were convinced, perhaps the researchers and the doubting parents would eventually be persuaded as well. But he needed a hook. A lure. An angle. He had Gloria, of course, but her story had already been told. One Williams person simply wasn't enough to be convincing. He needed more. He needed a phenomenon.

Howard remembered Lori Reyes from Hi Hopes. He was certain she had Williams syndrome; everyone had always joked about how much Lori and Gloria looked like sisters, and now he knew why. He approached her parents, explaining his goal of attracting researchers to study music and Williams syndrome. They were happy to help, if it would mean more chances for Lori to make music.

There was also piano player Tim Baley of Anaheim, another

Hi Hopes alumnus. As a boy, Tim took a battery of tests at a Denver mental hospital as doctors struggled to find a diagnosis for him beyond "retarded." There was one called the piano test; a tiny Tim was simply plopped before the keyboard, and doctors watched, pencils poised. Most kids smashed their hands down on the keys over and over again, but not Tim. He touched the keys tenderly, curiously, reverently. By the time Tim joined Hi Hopes, he was a polished concert pianist who had played for Liberace and had performed in nine countries.

Cathy Krieger was the daughter of Howard's colleagues at UCI. Cathy was born in Minneapolis and diagnosed with cerebral palsy when she was three, even though she had none of the symptoms. Her parents noticed that she mimicked singers with striking accuracy before she was five, then started picking out tunes on the piano and organ. She took up guitar in her teens, struggling mightily to get past the limits of her fine motor skills, and began writing her own songs. One was called, "Look At What Handicapped People Can Do," which declared, "We can sing, we can dance, we can even write stories too; / We can do the same things that all you people can do."

And there was Dennis Butcher, a rich baritone who played drums at a Sunday school for the developmentally disabled and attended a local college to learn independent-living skills. He was in a dance group at the Hi Hopes school, but wasn't yet in the band. Dennis, like Gloria, was obsessed with opera; they knew most every composer and plot twist and went to most every show mounted in Orange County. Afterward, they would haunt the stage doors for the chance to speak with the singers and say how much they enjoyed the performance.

And thus, the Williams Five was born. The band—Gloria, Dennis, Cathy, Tim, and Lori—practiced in the clubhouse of the Anaheim trailer park where Dennis's family lived. They treated rehearsals as parties, inviting kids to stop by and sing. Tim Baley's father was band director, and Howard took on the role of band manager with missionary zeal. Howard chose songs, booked senior centers and retirement villages—the same sort of places Hi Hopes had always played. Dennis's baritone and Gloria's soprano blended sweetly on duets like "For Always," made popular by Josh Groban and Lara Fabian, and Howard started calling them "the Jeanette MacDonald–Nelson Eddy of the Williams set." He called reporters from tiny local papers and convinced them to write stories about Williams syndrome and the band. He parlayed those clips into an ever larger press kit that he sent to ever larger papers to entice them to write.

Howard wanted impact. He wanted exposure. His vision was to have the Williams Five make its "world premiere" at the Williams Syndrome Association's national convention in San Diego in 1994. He called the Williams Syndrome Association, raved about the band's talent, and hoped they could be prominently featured and solidly supported. Howard had pitched the story to a reporter from the *Los Angeles Times*, and the *Times* was interested. He would need four handheld microphones, a mike for the piano, two stand mikes for the guitar and accordion, a cassette player hooked up to the sound system. . . .

Howard's fervor, association officials felt, left him a bit deluded. Frustration with him was growing deeper and deeper. The overwhelming majority of Williams children had no real musical talent, many in the association believed, and they were growing furious that Howard kept insisting otherwise. The national headquarters was juggling more and more phone calls from parents who resented all this harping on music, parents who saw no glimmer of musicality in their own children and were left to conclude there was something even *more* wrong with them. Many agreed that Williams people were drawn to music and loved hearing music; but they just didn't believe that Williams people were especially talented at making music. There just weren't thousands of Glorias out there, hiding under rocks, waiting to be discovered, and they didn't want every parent of a

Williams child to be expecting that he had a musical genius-in-waiting. It would be heartbreaking when they discovered the truth, and there was already so much heartbreak involved with raising a disabled child. The Williams Five could play at the banquet, Howard was told. During mealtime. That was it.

The Williams Syndrome Association had grown from 150 families to more than 2,500 families in less than a decade, and the conference was packed. As always, it started with the scientific symposium, and researchers were abuzz from the recent breakthroughs. "Building Bridges Across Disciplines: Cognition to Gene," the professional gathering was called, and it was hosted jointly by the Williams Syndrome Association, the Salk Institute, and the UCSD School of Medicine. The sessions pushed at the boundaries of what was known: "Williams Syndrome: A Window to the Architecture of Mind and Brain," "Dissociations in Higher Cognitive Functions in Williams Syndrome," and "New Methods of Brain Imaging: The Neural Basis of Williams Syndrome." And as always, the meetings for parents followed.

Association director Terry Monkaba was in the hotel bar with some other parents after the day's sessions had ended, enjoying the rousing repertoire of the resident pianist. Terry had fielded irate phone calls about Howard and his ideas about music, and she was sympathetic to those parents. But she also knew that it was martial music that inspired her son, Ben, to finally get up and walk at age four, and it was she who made sure the Williams Five would have its "world premiere" at the conference. She considered herself a neutral party in the Williams clan wars. Terry was enjoying a particularly bopping song by the resident pianist when she looked a little closer and realized the pianist wasn't a "resident" at all: She was actually one of the Williams people there for the conference. Her name was Amy Koch, she was in her twenties, and she had been playing by ear for as long as she could remember. Amy actually taught music in a preschool for a while. No, she wasn't being paid by the hotel; she just saw the silent piano and couldn't help herself. She loved playing music. It was one of her favorite things in the world.

Terry heard Howard's voice. She got a funny feeling. She would make sure that a grand piano was set up by the stage for the final night's performance, and that this latest Williams wonder, Amy Koch, would play after the Williams Five.

It was not ideal that the Williams Five's debut would take place during dinner, accompanied by the clink of silverware and the drone of dinner conversation. Howard hoped the *Los Angeles Times* reporter wouldn't find it too distracting. As the banquet plates emerged, the band took the stage and followed the program Howard had meticulously worked out: from "Something Beautiful" by Robbie Williams (Tim on piano, Lori and Dennis leading, Cathy and Gloria joining in for chorus) to a possible "Hokey Pokey" finale (a happy song to get everyone, especially little kids, clapping), with the "world premiere" of Cathy's original song, "A Better World," highlighted in the middle. That song was one of the best arguments for Howard's case: how many people with IQs in the fifty-five range could write original songs with lyrics that *rhyme*?

> Think of how wonderful this world would be,
> If everybody lived in peace and harmony.
> Well, I think that it would be a better world.
> Yes, I think that it would be a better world.

The Williams Five played with professionalism, undeterred by the din of diners. Children gathered at their feet, dancing wildly one minute, staring mesmerized at the performers the next. Howard's critics in the audience listened with what they considered open minds: the band was fine. Quite something, considering all the musicians had to work against one another. But honestly. They weren't heading for the top of the pop charts. The Williams Five was not stocked with Glorias.

After the band took its final bows and Howard fielded congratulations from many parents, Amy Koch sat down at the piano without hype or introduction. She played fluidly, gently, gracefully; some people didn't even listen. But Howard listened. To him, Amy's performance proved that musical talent was tied up with Williams syndrome. And Terry Monkaba listened as well. When the conference was over and Terry was back home in Michigan, the surprise discovery of Amy Koch weighed on her mind much more heavily than the appearance of the Williams Five.

For Howard, victory was sweet. "Beautiful Mystery; They Struggle to Tie Their Shoes and Make Change. But They Can Master Music and Languages. It's All Part of the Williams Syndrome Riddle," read the headline in the million-circulation *Los Angeles Times*. "Baley and his band-mates have Williams syndrome, a rare congenital disorder that has bolted from obscurity in the past few years to offer scientists a tantalizing riddle about the workings of the human mind," the story said. "How can the condition stunt most learning and intelligence but leave other complex skills, such as verbal abilities, unscathed or, seemingly, even enriched?"

Like a veteran politician, Howard stayed stubbornly on message, according to the article. "Lenhoff is eager for the scientific testing, which has so far dwelt on language abilities, to venture into the group's affinity for music. 'I can't wait,' he said. 'It is the aspect that fascinates me most . . . the connection with music is what makes Williams so different.'"

The reporter asked Lori what she would do without music, and she seemed unable to even comprehend the question. "What would I do without music? I don't know. I can't live without it," she said. "No songs? It would be . . . torment. Just torment."

"What is your secret wish?" the reporter asked.

"Well, I have always wanted to go on *Wheel of Fortune*," Lori said for a self-indulgent second. Then she veered back to her usual script and said emphatically, "I would want people to understand us. If people could see what we can do, all of us, what we can do as a person, then they would call us what we really are. Mentally gifted."

Howard tried to drive that point home as well. "How can we really say they are retarded or developmentally disabled?" he told the *Times*. "In many ways, some of these Williams kids are superior to a lot of typical people in verbal skills or music. I say the best thing to call them is mentally asymmetric. They are different, really. Not disabled."

The *Times* story catapulted Williams syndrome onto the national stage, and soon National Public Radio's *All Things Considered* called. Host Noah Adams, trying to learn to play piano at age forty, was intrigued by what he had read and wanted to do the story himself. Howard was thrilled. There was just one problem: The Williams Five had pretty much done already what it was designed to do. There were no more gigs scheduled. Undeterred, Howard simply got the band and the parents together in a conference room at UCI and let the NPR crew tape there.

The band members loved the attention. "I wish there was a class for people so they can learn exactly what it's like to be like this," Cathy told Adams, practically grabbing the microphone. "I mean, if people are going to laugh at us and tease us about a disability, they should go to a class and learn what it's like to have this thing. I mean, sometimes it's wonderful, but there are times when it's not a bundle of joy. You know, you want to be able to overcome all your fears, like of loud noises, and you struggle, and you struggle every day. . . . Sometimes it doesn't become better at all. You know, you struggle to become normal."

Adams was taken. "What can't you do on a daily basis that you would really like to do?"

Lori chimed in. "Can't get married, have a family, drive a car. Um, have a house," she said.

"Can you go shopping by yourself?" he asked.

"No," she said. "Because every time I go to a shopping mall, most of the time, I get lost. I get very lost. I get confused. I get disoriented. . . . Sometimes in a big restaurant it's hard for me to even find my way around. It's hard sometimes. You want to do something and you can't. And you get so frustrated."

Cathy jumped in. "What people need to understand is we're people like everybody else," she said. "We're just slower and do things differently than other people, that's all."

Dennis piped up. "I think a lot of people will be amazed to see like Gloria or Tim or Cathy or Lori or even me performing," he said. "You don't have to be ashamed to be a Williams syndrome. You have to love yourself and accept what God has given you to be in this world to live as a Williams syndrome."

Soon Howard got a call from a film student at the University of Southern California. Craig Detweiler was very different from the Hollywood elite he was training alongside; he had graduated from divinity school, was a devout Christian, and planned to make movies that spoke to the soul. He and his wife were making ends meet as night watchmen at a retirement home, but he was also doing some work for a Dutch production company. He took the *Los Angeles Times* article to them and said, "Doesn't this look interesting?" They gave him the go-ahead to do some research.

The first part of Howard's public relations offensive seemed to be succeeding wildly: Williams and music had clicked in the popular consciousness far beyond his expectations. Now he had to concentrate on the second part, the hardest part: getting the researchers to act.

Audrey Don had never heard of Gloria Lenhoff or Howard Lenhoff or the Williams Five. But before the *Los Angeles Times* and National Public Radio were doing stories on Williams syndrome, Don heard from her mentor that music and Williams syndrome might be linked. In her office in Ontario, Canada, she was trying to delve deeper.

Don was a neuropsychologist with an original bent. She had spent fifteen years working as a visual artist, creating prints and paintings, when she found herself volunteering at the local children's hospital doing art therapy with kids in the cancer ward. An eight-year-old girl with bone cancer was admitted and released several times; each time she returned to the hospital, she became more and more committed to becoming as fine an artist as she could be. The girl was amazed to watch her own skills develop, to actually be able to draw things that looked like she wanted them to look. It moved Don deeply to watch her grow artistically even as her body was failing. The girl fashioned an art gallery in her house and continued creating until the week before her death. Her artwork was her legacy, her parents said, the thing she was most proud of, the thing that made her feel she had accomplished something with her life, however short. It made Don think about the link between mind and matter, psychology and physiology. What was the physical root of things as abstract and intangible as emotions and talent?

Don soon abandoned the bohemian life in favor of a very different one: the life of an academic. She traded paintbrushes for textbooks and began doctorate studies in neuropsychology at the University of Windsor. Neuropsychology examines the relationship between the hardware (brain and nervous system) and the software (mental functions such as language, memory, and perception). It was born in the nineteenth century, when a French doctor named Paul Broca discovered the speech center of the brain by examining the remains of a man who had been able to understand language but had lost the ability to speak. His brain had suffered damage to the left frontal lobe, allowing Broca to surmise its function.

Don, once the avowed artist, began exhaustive studies of the anatomy, physiology, and pathology of the nervous system. The dryness of the science was a shock to her system. After weeks of memorizing the location and function of the frontal, parietal, temporal, and occipital lobes, Don craved a creative outlet. She had said all she needed to say with paint, and found herself gravitating toward music. She played viola as a child, and decided to start playing again. She found a teacher, and music reawakened something profound within her.

She first heard of Williams syndrome in passing in a neuropsychology class, where it was mentioned alongside other genetic syndromes and examples of atypical cognitive development, including savants. The autistic idiot savant was famous, thanks to Dustin Hoffman and *Rain Man*—otherwise low-functioning people who had one fantastical ability, like instantly calculating twelve-digit numbers in their heads or hearing complex music once and then playing it perfectly on piano. The word going around was that Williams might have its share of idiot savants, too.

Don was so enthralled by her reunification with the viola that she wanted to work music into her dissertation somehow. No one had investigated a link between Williams syndrome and music before; perhaps it was time to see if music should be added to the list of unusual Williams traits.

It was well accepted now that, somehow, verbal ability was relatively well preserved in Williams people. Don figured that if musical skills were also preserved, the two might be linked, and it probably had something to do with how the Williams brain processed auditory patterns. If the brain's machinery for processing and interpreting sound was somehow spared in Williams, it could help explain both abilities.

The Canadian Association for Williams Syndrome and the American Williams Syndrome Association helped Don find nineteen children between the ages of eight and thirteen. She would test them on verbal as well as musical abilities. She had never met Williams children before, and soon found herself with nineteen new friends whose affection sometimes seemed overenthusiastic, exaggerated, unregulated. Their need to connect and interact emotionally with other people was striking; it seemed to nourish them. It was very curious.

First Don looked at language and spatial skills. She knew to expect an abyss between the children's performance on the verbal and spatial tests, but she was still astounded by the greatness of the gap in abilities. But more subtle and more interesting to her was the clear hierarchy within their celebrated verbal abilities. The more complex the task, Don found, the worse the children did. On the simplest test—which asked them to recognize patterns of words broken into phonemes (bat, cat, mat, rat)—they performed close to normal for children their age, a tremendous feat considering their disabilities. But when asked to do the most complex tasks—verbal comprehension, understanding the meanings behind words, sentences, and paragraphs—the Williams children scored far below the mean for children their age. Their language skills weren't all they had been touted to be.

Then she went to the heart of her project. Were Williams kids exceptionally musical? She tested for tonal skills and rhythm skills, using Gordon's Primary Measures of Music Audiation, a test developed by a music educator with a master's degree in string bass performance. "Audiation" is simply the ability to hear music in one's head, much as he might see a picture in his mind's eye. The tests required no reading or music skills, just musical memory. They could be done in twenty-two-minute blocks of time, short enough to keep the attention of most Williams kids. The results would show what happened when the kids "heard" music through recall, when sound wasn't physically present. Based on what she had heard, she was expecting strong performances.

The tonal test was simple: one electronically generated melody, followed closely by another. The child had to say whether those melodies were the same or different. There were forty pairs of these.

The rhythm test was similar. One pattern would play, then another. Some were short, some were long. The child had to say whether the patterns were the same or different. There were forty of these as well.

Don traveled all over Ontario and the northeastern seaboard of the United States testing her subjects. The results surprised her. The Williams children did well, but not spectacularly well, and certainly not "idiot savant" well. And to Don's surprise, they did better with melody than with rhythm: Their mean tonal score was at the sixty-eighth percentile, about the same as a control group of "regular" children matched for language skills. But the Williams kids' mean rhythm score was at the forty-eighth percentile, lower than the regular children.

All told, her work showed that music skills in children with Williams were about as strong as their relatively preserved verbal skills—far better than one might expect, but not quite normal, and certainly not extraordinary.

But Don felt there was more going on. So she went beyond the numbers to do something much more subjective and potentially quite revealing: a "child music interest survey." It asked parents how much their children enjoyed music, what sort of musical activities they did, the environment at home, and how many sounds the kids could identify. She surveyed regular kids as well as the Williams group.

Here, the differences were tremendous. Williams children responded to music far more viscerally than the regular children did, she found: a full 100 percent of Williams kids said music could make them feel happy, compared to 84 percent of regular kids.

An overwhelming 79 percent of Williams kids said music could make them feel sad, compared to just 47 percent of regular kids. Two of the Williams kids said music was such an intense emotional experience that they had a love/hate relationship with it. And several parents offered, without being asked, that, as babies, their children screamed or cried uncontrollably when they heard beautiful lullabies or slow, relaxing songs, much as Gloria had when she heard Brahms's "Lullaby" as an infant. The Williams kids were also moved to tears by music far more often than regular kids were. "That music was so beautiful I couldn't listen to it anymore," one child said.

This is where the Williams kids' facility with language made Don's job fascinating. They could tell her exactly what in the music so moved them. One kid said it was the "don't leave me" songs that made her lose control. Another it was the mournful wailing of the violin. And one said something that she would never forget: "Music is my favorite way of thinking."

After all was said and done, Don concluded that Williams wasn't a savant mystery after all. Williams people were simply completely captivated by music, much more so than typical children. From the neuropsychologist's perspective, this made sense. Their hyperresponsiveness was probably connected to their hypersensitivity to sound, which led to extreme emotional responses. They had greater awareness of sound than regular kids, paid more attention to music than regular kids, responded more passionately than regular kids. It didn't seem that they were, as a group, any more talented than regular kids; but it made sense that their passion for music might lead them to develop relatively good musical skills. When you have the interest, you have the pathway to develop skills, Don said.

"The present study is the first to provide compelling empirical evidence that music skills represent areas of relative strength for children with WS," Don and her colleagues wrote in *Child Neuropsychology*. "[But] musicality in children with WS may stand out in some instances to clinicians, parents, and teachers because of its relative strength, rather than because of high, absolute or savant-like levels of skill. . . .

"The enthusiasm and emotional responsivity to music demonstrated by [Williams] children . . . combined with their relatively intact music abilities, raises the possibility that purposeful development of musical skills could help to enrich the lives of these children."

So much, she thought, could be done with this.

{chapter 9}

THE MUSIC CAMP EXPERIMENT

here was some tension. But in the end, the Williams Syndrome Association embraced the Belvoir Terrace music camp idea, though not without caveats. Camp was for the amusement of the children, not for the sake of serious study, the association stressed.

Howard smiled tightly and thanked the association for its support. If he had to bite his tongue so the camp could be publicized by the association—now reaching nearly three thousand families—he'd do it. But in truth, he, Sharon, and Nancy hoped that camp would indeed spark serious study. Their dearest wish was to ignite hidden potential in the kids, to inspire their parents to become forceful advocates, to send every last camper scrambling for serious music lessons upon returning home.

The registration deadline came and went. Of all the Williams Syndrome Association's members, only thirty-nine signed up—and Howard and Sharon worried that some of them wouldn't even show. Nancy wanted fifty campers so she stood a chance of breaking even. Eleven short. Howard and Sharon worried that, after all this work, Nancy would call the whole thing off.

They held their breath as they told Nancy about the low

enrollment. Nancy shrugged and changed the subject. Her curiosity had been so piqued by the charm of John Libera and the power of Gloria's voice that she decided the camp would simply work, somehow or other, end of story. It would begin the week after regular camp ended with a staff of nearly eighty. Excitedly, Sharon wrote press releases and sent them to every media outlet she could think of: "The nation's first camp for mentally disadvantaged children and adults who show a gift for music and the arts will open this summer. . . ." it began. It ended with a quote from Howard: "This camp is just the beginning. My dream goes beyond, to the establishment of a residential music and arts college for the nation's artistically-gifted, mentally disadvantaged."

When a few local reporters started calling and asking to visit, Williams Syndrome Association director Terry Monkaba found herself trying to dampen sky-high expectations. You are *not* going to find a camp full of Gloria Lenhoffs here, she told them. These kids love music, but they are not prodigies.

The night before camp began, Howard, Sharon, and Nancy huddled with the entire Belvoir staff, like generals in a war room with the entire army; so many of the staffers were so young. Gloria sang an aria. Howard gave them an overview of the genetics and science. Sharon gave them a crash course on what Williams people were like: distractible, extremely sensitive to criticism, poor at concepts and spatial skills, hypersensitive to sound, disturbed by changes in routine, insecure on open stairs, and the like. They were also very friendly, learned well when praised, imitated easily, liked structure and knowing what was going to happen next. Nancy gave two commands: know where the campers are at all times, and teach by rote. Williams kids were not able to think logically or solve problems, but they could practice the same thing over and over until they knew it. They found repetition engrossing, not boring, so repeat, repeat, repeat. It was the direct opposite of everything the teachers had always striven for.

They all agreed on one rule: no research was to be done while camp was in session. Scientists investigating health, personality, and cognition might want to capitalize on having so many Williams people together in one place, but it would not be allowed. Camp was for the kids, not for the researchers. If scientists wanted subjects for a study, they could ask that families come a day earlier or stay a day later. But camp itself was not to be disturbed.

The next day, Bob Ackley made the turn onto Greenwood Street while his daughter, Tori, looked eagerly out the car window. When Tori was six, she started playing songs on her toy telephone, picking out "Mary Had a Little Lamb" with the tones on the keypad. When Bob spotted the grand mansion on the hill and saw its sprawling front lawn, he started crying. My baby's going *here*?! he said to himself as he pulled up the long driveway.

Nancy's mother, Edna Schwartz, sat in a purple golf cart, dressed in a purple shirt, purple pants, and a purple hat, waving him on and shouting, "This way!" Bob followed her all the way up the mansion's gravel drive, where Nancy waited with a clipboard.

Over the decades, Nancy had developed an MO for the first day of camp. She'd stand in the drive as parents arrived with their girls so she could see returning campers bolt from still-rolling cars to hop and squeal and seize friends they hadn't seen since the summer before. She'd also witness the tears and the trepidation of the new girls as they arrived, knowing no one, afraid of spending their first summer away from their families. It never failed to be a poignant and uproarious slice of life.

But as Nancy stood there to greet the Williams campers, she saw a spectacle that outdid anything she had witnessed before. It was feverish, ecstatic entropy. Children who had never met shrieked and hugged and hung on one another like long-lost loves; they glad-handed from adult to adult, excitedly confessing how happy they were to be there and how wonderful it was to meet you and how they had never been to camp before and wasn't this just so thrilling and they already wished it would never end. Often, Williams people were riddled with anxiety when entering new social situations; they wanted so much to be liked and to fit in, and they worried so much about rejection. But here, they seemed to know that they all were safe, that they all belonged. Nancy was not a sappy woman, but even she found a knot growing in her throat as she watched them come together, like the members of a long-forgotten tribe. She couldn't believe how much they looked alike, more like one another than like their own parents, in many cases. It was so strange.

As Howard watched, he felt, for a moment, a deep satisfaction. It was, in so many ways, a dream coming true right before his eyes. But that serenity was quickly followed by a jolt of adrenaline and a plaintive prayer: please, please, let the rest of the week go well. If something goes wrong, we'll never hear the end of it.

Seized by the spirit of exploration, Gloria and the campers raided the stone mansion to investigate their new digs. Spirited choruses of "Wow!" erupted as the campers gawked at the mansion's soaring ceilings, the massive stone fireplace, and the beauty of the green, rolling hills through the giant windows. Chris Lawson, eighteen, headed straight for the piano and played "The Australian Ladies," a mournful song that, he explained apologetically, he usually played on bagpipes. Others crowded around to listen. His long, thin fingers seemed to encompass whole tracts of the keyboard and it was hard to pry him away; he launched into military marches, the theme from *Love Story*, and on and on. Gloria broke away to introduce herself to her counselor and her teachers, wanting to know who'd be teaching her what and where and when. It was cheerful chaos.

The investigation progressed to the woodsy dormitory, a dark, low-slung two-story building behind the mansion. Boys on the top floor, girls on the bottom. Gloria's little room brimmed with bunk beds, smelled of wood and dust, and echoed faintly with decades of late-night whispers and schoolgirl secrets. The room had bunks for eight—four Williams girls on the bottom, four counselors (to keep an eye on them) up top—all covered with dark wool blankets despite the summer heat, because it got cold at night in the Berkshires. Many of the counselors were former Belvoir campers who volunteered in exchange for room, board, and the chance to return to the camp they so loved.

Cathy Krieger, who sang with Gloria in the Williams Five, was one of Gloria's roommates, as was Anne Louise McGarrah, the woman she met at the Boston convention in 1990. Anne learned piano as a girl, but she hadn't played for some thirty years and was looking forward to rediscovering her music. They compared notes as they unpacked, stuffing their things into cubbyholes and stashing suitcases under beds, feeling as if they were on a true adventure.

Campers ranged in age from nine to forty-six, and their first official activity was dinner in the long, long dining room. Nancy used all the volume she could muster to quiet the campers down and explain what would be happening over the next week; she had learned that they liked to know what was happening next. The days would be carved into several periods, she said—instrumental lessons, musical theater, movement—and the campers would have to change locations each period. A counselor would escort them from place to place to avoid confusion. Meals would be served "family-style," and whoever sat at the head of the table was responsible for going to the food window, gathering up bowls of meat and vegetables and potatoes, and transporting it all back to the table intact, where bowls would pass from person to person and back again. Each table had to clean up its own mess—there weren't any maids here. There'd be different activities every night—campfires and talent shows and faculty recitals—and she hoped everyone would participate and have a ball. On the very last night of camp, there would be a special grand finale show, and people from all over town would be invited. Pay attention in those dance and musical theater classes, she told them.

That night, there was a campfire. Flames crackled and hissed and threw clouds of gold and orange light through the dark woods. Children and parents and staffers gathered around it, sitting on soggy logs as decaying leaves were mushed underfoot, cooking chocolate-and-marshmallow s'mores in the fire, singing "This Land Is Your Land" while Gloria played accordion. Many of the kids couldn't contain themselves and leapt to their feet to dance, shimmying around the fire like warriors in some raucous ritual.

There were twenty-five moms and dads at camp, and they agreed to watch the dorms while the counselors got a break between 9 and 11 PM. They stood outside in the cold night air, the sky so bright and clear you could see the Milky Way, and listened. Lights snapped off at 10 PM, but that didn't stop the excited chatter: bunkmates chronicled hometowns and schools and favorite bands, professed that they'd be friends forever, and said they couldn't wait to see what would happen tomorrow. At home, Williams kids didn't have confidantes and friendships like this. Here, suddenly, was an instant community.

At breakfast the next day, the children greeted one another as if they had been apart for years. Wordplay was a common game: "It's A-OK at the KOA!" a camper joked. An exclamation of "Funky!" inspired rounds of "Spunky to your monkey to your donkey!" And a discussion of perfect pitch lead to rapperlike riffing on "pitch, witch, stitch, rich, hitch, ditch." Then the campers headed off to their first lessons, often clinging to the arms of their escorts.

There were two kinds of classes: large classes for chorus, dance, and musical theater; and small ones for instrument lessons.

Chorus was held in an airy studio with high ceilings, a honey-colored floor, and tremendous half-moon windows resembling giant Chinese fans that washed the room with sunlight. A teacher played "The Lion Sleeps Tonight" on violin and the entire group grabbed drums and shakers and tambourines and rhythm sticks and triangles and joined in, dancing riotously.

An open-air studio on a hill surrounded by verdant green was the setting for dance classes, and some of the kids were so excited they pretended to be ballerinas pirouetting wildly across the floor. Reach up, up, up to the sky, like you're trying to milk a very tall cow, teachers said as kids giggled. Line up and prance cross the floor! The campers did as they were told, but only what they were told: when they got to the other side of the room, they didn't turn around and come back to their starting places, as the teachers expected. They simply stood there, facing the wall, until they were told to turn around and return. Williams kids did follow directions explicitly—but they had to be extremely explicit, providing the finest details. The kids simply could not logically divine the next step in an exercise, even if it seemed painfully obvious to others.

Bryce Hill, the musical theater teacher, had met Gloria and John Libera before camp started, and expected to see that kind of high-end talent in the rest of the campers. That was clearly not the case. His charge was to whip up mini-musicals in a week, which would be performed in the grand finale on the closing night of camp: *The Wizard of Oz* for the younger kids, *Pippin* for the older kids, and *Grease* for the adults, like Gloria. He noticed that the teenage girls tended to take over and grab the limelight, singing and dancing with no inhibitions whatsoever, while the boys hung back unsteadily. Bryce was having trouble getting the boys to sing. He was racking his brain trying to figure out how to get them to participate when they all professed to have expertise with some instrument or other—trombone, trumpet, clarinet.

OK, Bryce said. Let's try that. He was not feeling very optimistic as the instruments came out of their cases. But when the pianist started playing, the boys started honking and bleeping along. Not from sheet music, but by ear and from sheer memory. It was rough. It was bumpy. But the guts of the song were there. That's when the little light went on inside Bryce's head; as long as we keep raising the bar, he thought, these kids are going to keep clearing it. So he improvised, gathering everyone around the piano and singing the parts they needed to learn to make the musical work; he found it only took one or two tries before the campers had everything memorized.

The intimate music lessons were a different story. They were held in small practice rooms scattered along the hillsides, and took the "first date" approach: the aim was to give the campers a fun and pleasant introduction to the instruments, not to expect accomplishment. One of the instrumental teachers was Nancy's daughter Laura, who taught chamber music and violin in the Juilliard School's precollege program. Chamber music, however, was far too advanced for this crowd, and the violin was far too difficult for most Williams kids to handle. Instead, Laura would teach guitar.

Laura had never taught developmentally disabled students before. She knew that most Williams people had problems with fine motor coordination, as well as joint problems that caused abnormalities in their hands and wrists. She knew they couldn't read music. So she tuned the guitars to an open G major chord. Then, by simply pressing a finger—or pencil or pen or whatever was handy—across the entire neck of the guitar, then sliding it up or down, campers could made different chords and play songs. With shaky fingers and yellow pencils stretched across guitar necks, campers plunked out "Feeling Groovy," "You Are My Sunshine," and simple folk songs that made them shriek, "I'm making music!" Most campers seemed to know the words by heart and sang along—on-key, off-key, and occasionally very off-key—strumming with abandon and, sometimes, nearly the proper rhythm. This style of guitar class was dropped in later years—guitar is notoriously difficult for many Williams people to play—but in all her years of teaching, Laura had never seen people get so excited over music. It didn't matter if they were good or not. It didn't matter if they were playing or hearing someone else play. Their reactions were bigger, stronger, and

more dramatic than anything she had encountered. Their enjoyment was more intense and passionate than anything she had
experienced.

In the private voice lessons, Gloria worked on her enunciation in Italian: "Meeeee ahhhhh, like Mia Farrow, the ahhhhhh-
hhhhhhs very bright, lots of light. . . . Your 'la' is not as wonderful as it can be. Can you make it more wonderful? A very
lively ahhhhh. . . ." John Libera's piano teacher showed him the
trick of scooting his thumb behind his pinky to smoothly move
down the keyboard while playing. In another class, John picked
up a clarinet for the first time, fell in love with its expressive,
almost-human voice, and was playing songs by the end of his first
lesson. It became apparent to the teachers that Gloria, John, and
many of the other campers had perfect pitch, the ability to hear a
single, solitary note and to know it is a G, or an A, or a B-flat. It
was a rare ability, even among musicians.

Nancy was in the practice rooms watching her great experiment unfold as the children wrestled with drumsticks and saxophones for the first time. She watched them in dance class, in
musical theater, in performance. She almost always had a video
camera in her hands and she saw things that only a longtime
teacher could see. There was not a great deal of accomplishment
in this crowd—not at all. But there was a great deal of aptitude.
Raw material. Interest that could be harnessed, shaped, refined.
Passion always precedes accomplishment, she felt. And in this
crowd, there was a staggering amount of passion.

Consider Alec Sweazy. He was only nine. Thin and reedy,
mischievous and fidgety, with a mushroom cap of bouncy blond
hair and otherworldly eyes—the blue of glaciers, patterned like
ice that has fissured and fractured. His irises were shot through
with lacy star patterns—one telltale sign of the syndrome. Alec
was the mysteriously musical infant who sang tones back to his
mother, on pitch, when he was not yet three months old. Now,
Alec could copy everything the teachers showed him on piano

and was ravenous to play every instrument he could lay his hands on. He became enamored of Gloria's accordion, and she was soon giving him lessons; they sat, young boy and grown woman, threading their arms through the ungainly instruments, as Gloria showed him how to pump bellows and squeeze buttons to coax the instrument's carnival voice to life.

And there was Brian Johnson. He was singing along to Kenny Rogers songs before he spoke sentences; when he was five, his grandmother bought him a piano just because she had always wanted someone in the family to play. His mother was his first teacher, playing a note and saying, This is a G . . . this is a D . . . this is an A. . . . Brian would inevitably get bored and retreat to the sofa. His mom would continue striking keys—This is an F, this is a B—until one day he said, No, Mom. That's not a B. That's a C. It startled her. He was right. She played notes and asked him to name them. *A. D. E.* She was surprised by his accuracy. She played chords; he named all the notes that made up the chords. He's possessed! she and his father thought. In fact, what he had was perfect pitch. When Brian had trouble in school, his mother sang his homework to him to help him grasp it more easily.

Brian had picked up the guitar a few years ago, figured out the open-tuning trick that Laura Goldberg was using in guitar class, and discovered the elation of singing. His was a husky voice, almost Dylanesque, and he studied with a jazz vocalist at a North Carolina community college, sometimes sitting in on Tuesday night gigs at Amos' Bar and Bistro. Brian was particularly partial to "Ain't Misbehavin'," knew the lyrics to an exhaustive number of pop songs, could quickly weave harmonies, and was constantly making up his own songs in the shower, while doing homework, when cleaning up his room. His parents followed him around with tape recorders and video cameras to capture the music as it surged out of him; he could not write it down, and they didn't want it to lose it.

There was Chris Lawson, with his lyric hands and his Scottish bagpiper's cap. In addition to his skill on piano, he was a lead drummer for the Stuart Highlanders Pipe Band in Connecticut and performed in parades in New England. There was Tori Ackley, only ten, a devotee of Raffi. There was Anne McGarrah, at the keyboard for the first time in decades, playing pieces she had learned thirty years before.

On the third night of camp, they all squished into a music lounge, sat knee to knee on the floor, and remained there, transfixed, for nearly three hours as each camper took a turn in the spotlight. It didn't seem to matter if it was as simple as playing air guitar to a tape recording or as complicated as singing an aria or as lengthy as a full rendition of "American Pie"; their attention and enthusiasm never flagged, even when the performances were downright terrible. They cheered, they clapped, they hooted and hollered, they danced and rocked and gave each other high fives. Anne McGarrah jumped up with the passion of a preacher and whipped everyone into a frenzy: "Look what we have! We have talent here! We have L-O-V-E! We have F-R-I-E-N-D-S-H-I-P! Are we going to let the fact that we have a birth defect ruin our lives? No!"

Nancy invited cellist Yo-Yo Ma out to Belvoir to take a look. Gloria sang for him and was thrilled when he kissed her cheek. Tanglewood Music Festival voice coach Alan Townsend also visited and helped Gloria with her enunciation of some Italian words. Boston Pops conductor Keith Lockhart welcomed campers to a rehearsal of the orchestra as well, and he was as wowed as Nancy at how obviously entranced the campers were by the music.

Nancy wanted other people to experience these campers, who were so vastly different from the kind of kids she was used to. Nancy's regulars were always so concerned about how they appeared before others; they'd never get up in front of a crowd and perform if they didn't know their piece very, very well. But

the Williams campers didn't care at all. They didn't get stage
fright. They couldn't be embarrassed. And, more strikingly,
most didn't seem to have a trace of envy or jealousy. They were
genuinely generous of spirit, supporting one another enthusiastically, joyously, wholeheartedly, with their raucous whooping
and cheering. It melted Nancy's heart. She had never seen anything like it.

Belvoir's tradition was to hold the grand finale under the hot
stage lights on the last night, showing off the campers' accomplishments before a sympathetic audience of parents and neighbors. This show was going to be rougher than the usual Belvoir
fare, Nancy knew, but she couldn't wait to see it.

All thirty-nine campers were in the theater early, dabbing
their faces with powder and running through scales in unison.
When the house lights dimmed and the stage lights rose, a chorus
line of the smallest campers took the stage, giggling and wiggling,
and bleated through songs from *The Wizard of Oz*: "Somewhere
over the Rainbow," "Ding Dong the Witch Is Dead," and "We're
Off to See the Wizard." They sang at the top of their lungs, more
funny than fab, not at all concerned with hitting the right notes,
and when they were done they leaped in the air and howled with
joy. Then the older campers took the stage, adorned in tree tinsel,
singing songs from *Pippin* with similar abandon; and then the
adults came on stage—men in jeans and T-shirts, women in
poodle skirts and sweaters—to sing songs from *Grease*. Gloria's
soaring soprano lent a peculiar dimension to "Summer Loving,"
"Look at Me, I'm Sandra Dee," and "We Go Together," but the
other Williams folks, as always, roared with approval.

It was not an accomplished program. Often, it was an occasionally painful take on amateur night. But the campers were
having a wonderful time and clearly loved music more than anything; they were enormous hams, adoring stage and spotlight
and, especially, microphone. It was a testament to the generosity

of their spirits that they sat there, rapt, through each piece, receiving every performer as if he or she was one of the Beatles. But some in the audience just couldn't escape the conclusion that the overwhelming majority lacked not only any hint of accomplishment, but also any glimmer of raw talent. As everyone rose in a standing ovation, Howard couldn't stop talking about all the potential he saw; some of the parents looked at him with awe, wondering if they had seen the same show he saw. Were they on the same planet?

After the last howls of appreciation died down and Howard thanked Sharon for her vision and Nancy for her hard work, Sharon took the stage.

"I went for a walk in this beautiful natural setting and found this," she said, holding up a tiny object. "Do you know what this is?"

"*An acorn!*" the campers thundered.

"It will turn into a big tree and have beautiful leaves and apples and all the fruit you can eat!" one girl yelled.

Sharon smiled. "Yes, it's an acorn, and this acorn reminded me of Howard Lenhoff," she said. The campers found that hilarious. "From the seed of Gloria's ability, he helped her grow, and then didn't just keep it in his own family; he looked around and saw what was possible for the rest of us. He saw something small, and is growing something very big."

She handed him the acorn, and he held onto it as if it were a jewel. Then he pulled out a sack of trophies, each inscribed with a camper's name and the words "Belvoir Star," which was Sylvia's inspiration. The children paraded on stage, one by one, and grabbed the awards with excitement worthy of Grammy winners. Association director Terry Monkaba, who was still trying to juggle the demands of the various parental factions, made a mental note to buy her son Ben—who had been banging on desk and tabletops with his pencils for as long as she could remember—a drum set.

What many campers called the best week of their lives was over. They had never had so much fun before. They had never had so many friends before. Many cried as they packed their things and loaded their cars, vowing to never forget one another and to stay in touch and to always be friends.

I loved it more than anything, Cathy Krieger said. Nobody teased me. It was so comfortable.

John Libera turned to Sharon and asked, Can we stay here forever? Sharon's heart melted.

What about Dad? she asked.

Well, we can have him come out too, John offered.

Nancy was already certain she'd be hosting the Williams camp again next year. She saw past the off-key singing and the laborious piano playing and the honking saxophones that tripped up the skeptics to something deeper. Music lived inside these kids. She felt certain of it. It was in them to a much greater degree than she had seen in any other group. They could listen to music longer than any others she had ever known. They could hear it and know it and, it seemed, never forget it. Nancy had lots of experience with truly gifted musicians—Yo-Yo Ma, Itzhak Perlman—and in her opinion, they were all a little odd. Wonderfully odd. None of them were good at ordinary things. They had business managers who wrote their letters and wives who drove them around and assistants who kept their calendars. They didn't worry about what they looked like or if they combed their hair or brushed their teeth—they were essentially on another planet. Planet Music, if you will. They heard music all the time. In their heads. And Nancy was sure that a lot of the Williams kids heard music in their heads, too.

"It's as if one part of the brain is not functioning while another part is overfunctioning," she told a local newspaper, trying to make sense of what she had seen.

Nancy and her staff did for the Williams campers exactly what they did for the regular campers: reviewed the performance of each child and sent letters home with specific recommendations on how parents should nurture their child's abilities. Tori, Nancy said, needed singing and piano lessons. Alec needed to buckle down on the keyboard. John Libera was obviously enthralled with the clarinet and should add that instrument to his lesson list. And so on and so on, for all thirty-nine campers. Nancy had spent enough time around kids to know that the most talented children invariably had the most driven parents; you get out what you put in, she told them. That was obviously the case with the Lenhoffs and Gloria, with the Liberas and John, and it was true with all children, handicapped or not. The younger you start them, the better they'll be. And don't just make sure they practice every day; practice with them.

When all the letters were out and Nancy was closing down the mansion for the winter, she had the overwhelming feeling that she had been part of something truly extraordinary, truly earthshaking. They are the most beautiful people I have ever met, her daughter Diane said. Nancy wholeheartedly agreed.

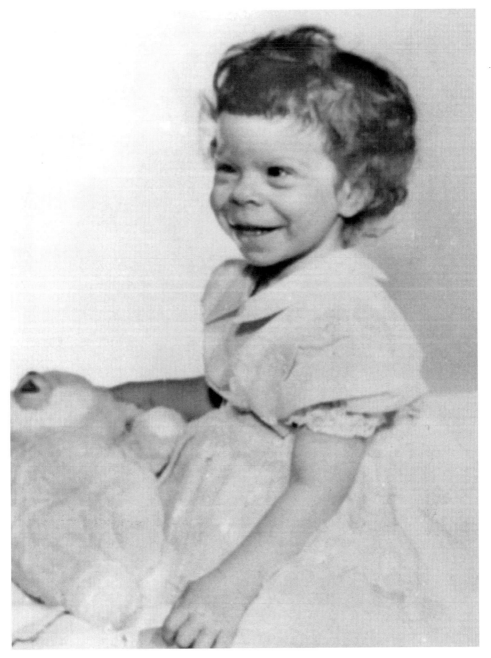

Gloria, as a toddler, smiled easily for photographers and other strangers.
Photo courtesy of the Lenhoff family.

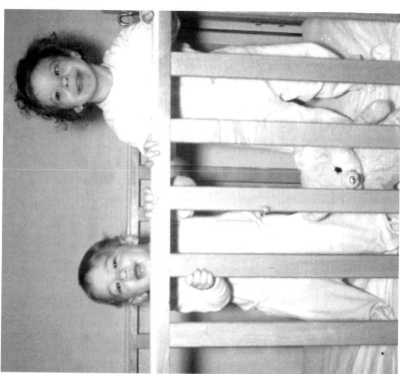

Little brother Bernie and big sister Gloria were playmates as babies, and Bernie was a good developmental role model for Gloria in Washington, DC, May 1958. *Photo courtesy of the Lenhoff family.*

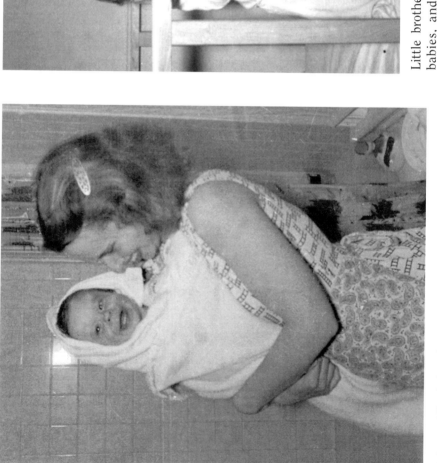
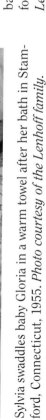

Sylvia swaddles baby Gloria in a warm towel after her bath in Stamford, Connecticut, 1955. *Photo courtesy of the Lenhoff family.*

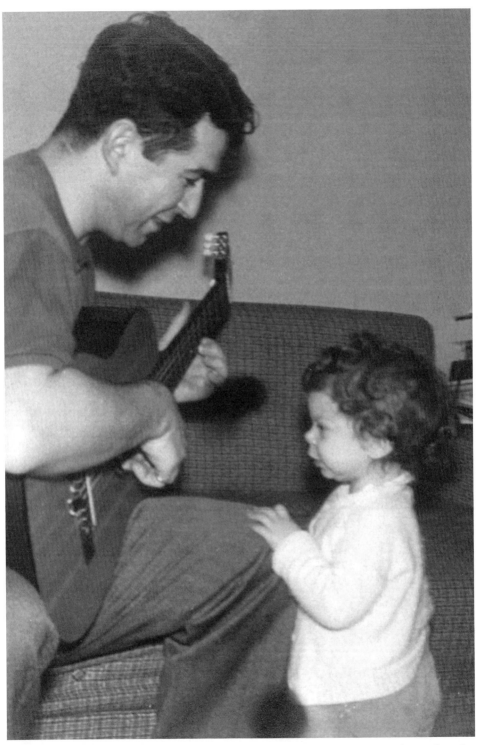

When Howard played his classical guitar, Gloria snapped to attention and stared at the strings, mesmerized. *Photo courtesy of the Lenhoff family.*

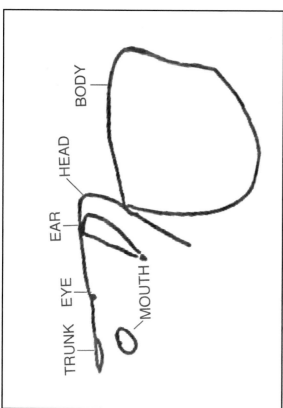

People with Williams syndrome have great difficulties with visual and spatial thinking. Dr. Ursula Bellugi of the Salk Institute for Biological Studies in San Diego asked a teenager with Williams to draw an elephant. This very rudimentary drawing stood in striking contrast to the teen's poetic description of the elephant, detailing its "long, gray ears, fan ears, ears that can blow in the wind." *Photo courtesy of Dr. Ursula Bellugi, The Salk Institute, La Jolla, CA.*

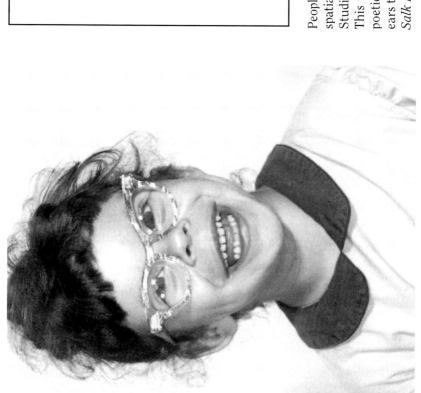

Gloria enjoys getting her school picture taken, around second grade, at Dade Elementary, Coral Gables, Florida. *Photo courtesy of the Lenhoff family.*

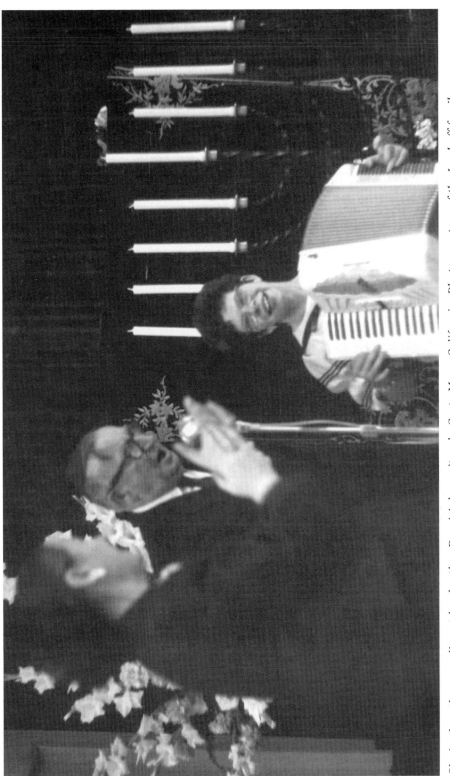

Gloria plays the accordion at her brother Bernie's bar mitzvah, Costa Mesa, California. *Photo courtesy of the Lenhoff family.*

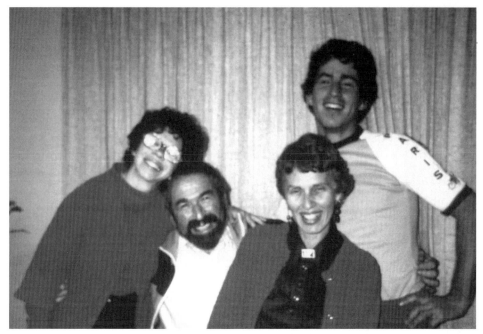

The Lenhoffs pose for a family portrait in their Costa Mesa home in 1981. *Photo courtesy of the Lenhoff family.*

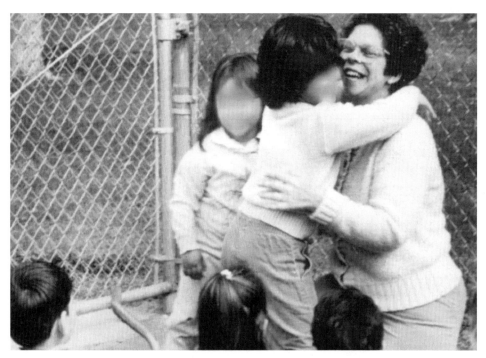

Hugs were one of the best parts of the job when Gloria volunteered at a daycare center in Orange, California, in 1986. *(Children's faces obscured to protect privacy.) Photo by Arlene Alda.*

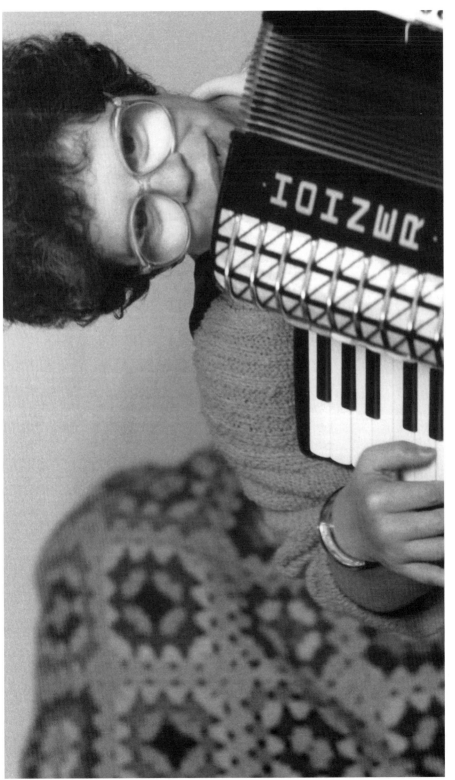

Gloria concentrates on making music during the shooting of the documentary *Bravo, Gloria! Photo by Arlene Alda.*

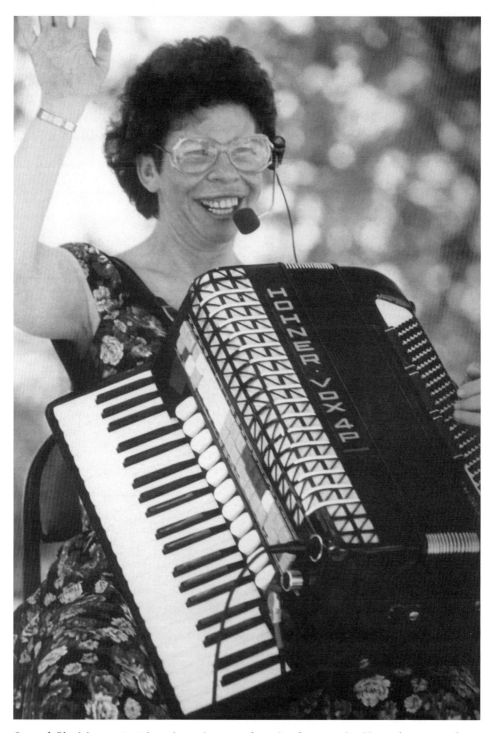

One of Gloria's greatest joys is seeing people enjoy her music. Here she responds to applause at a performance for UCI students during its "disability week" in October 1991. *Photo courtesy of the Lenhoff family.*

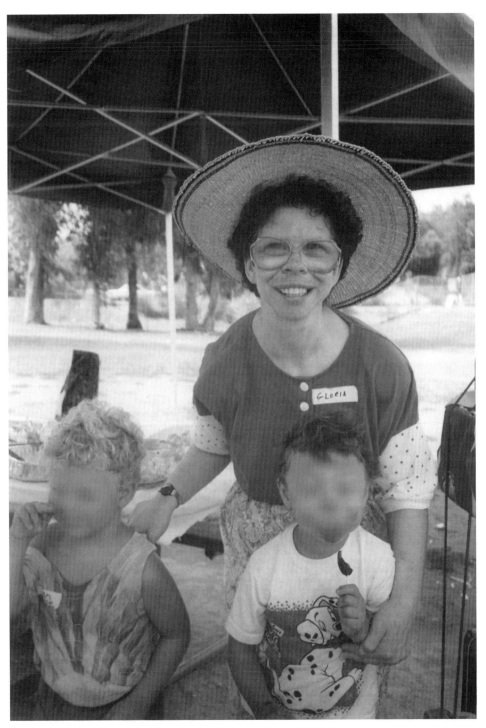

Gloria keeps an eye on children at a Williams Syndrome Association picnic in San Diego in 1991. Their simple exuberance was always something she could relate to. *Photo courtesy of the Lenhoff family.*

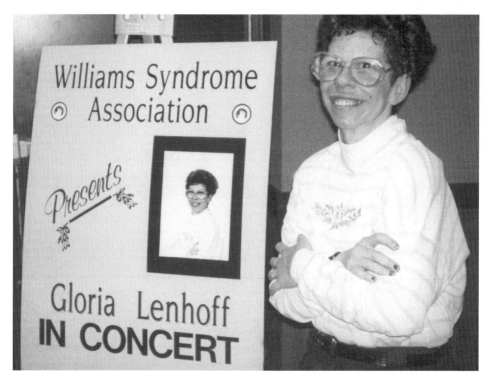

In the early days, the Lenhoffs attended conferences of the Williams Syndrome Association so Gloria could have a place to perform and inspire other Williams families. *Photo courtesy of the Lenhoff family.*

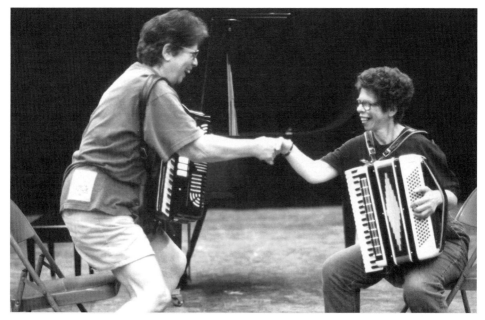

Belvoir Terrace camp director Nancy Goldberg (left) shakes Gloria's hand after a rousing accordion duet. *Photo courtesy of Belvoir Terrace.*

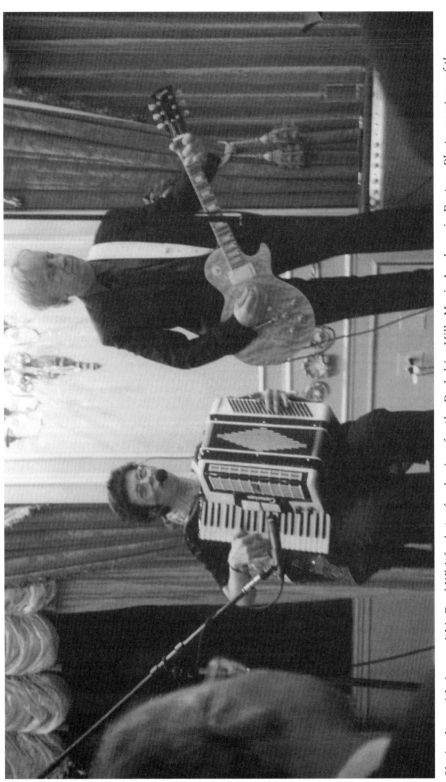

Gloria plays with Aerosmith's Brad Whitford at a fund-raiser for the Berkshire Hills Music Academy in Boston. *Photo courtesy of the Lenhoff family.*

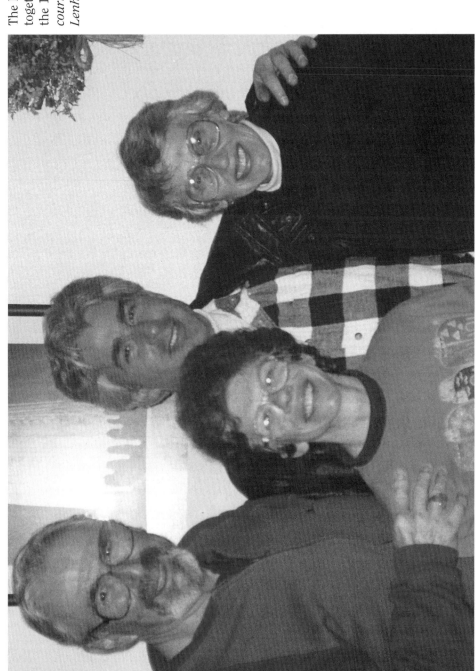

The Lenhoff family, together again in the 1990s. *Photo courtesy of the Lenhoff family.*

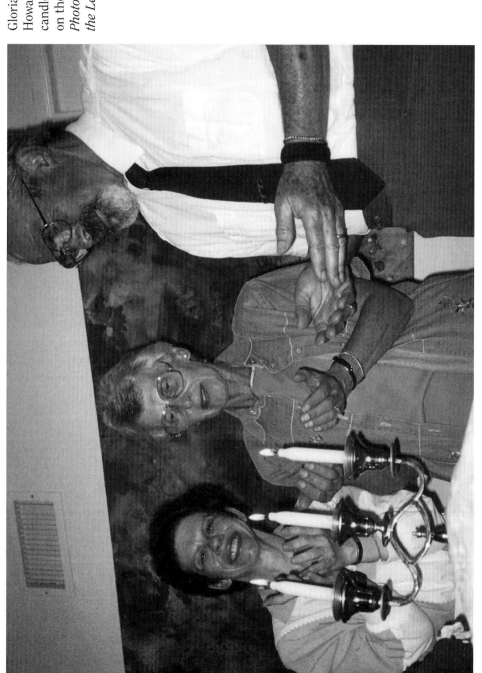

Gloria, Sylvia, and Howard light candles together on the Sabbath. *Photo courtesy of the Lenhoff family.*

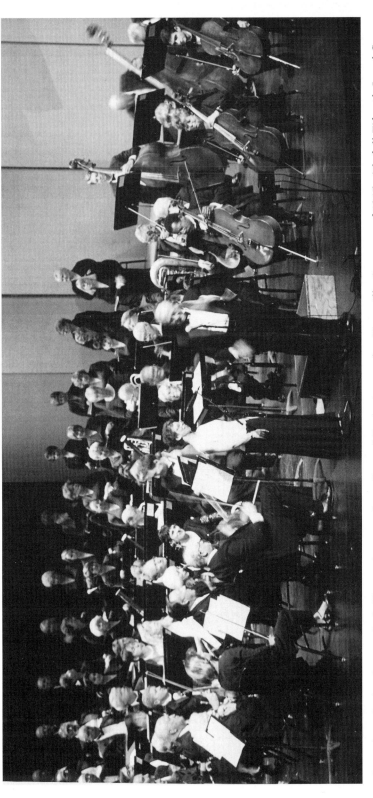

Gloria does the hardest work she'd ever done: perform Samuel Barber's complex *Knoxville, Summer of 1915* with full Tifereth Israel Community Orchestra in San Diego County. *Photo courtesy of the Lenhoff family.*

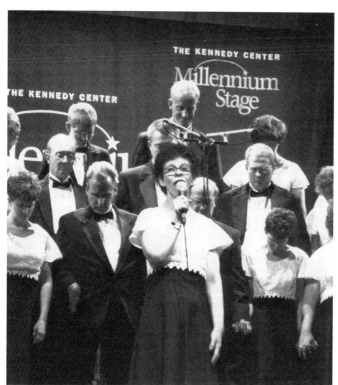

Gloria sings "The Lord's Prayer" at the Kennedy Center's Millennium Stage as the Baddour Center's Miracles choir joins hands behind her. *Photo courtesy of Pamela Antill.*

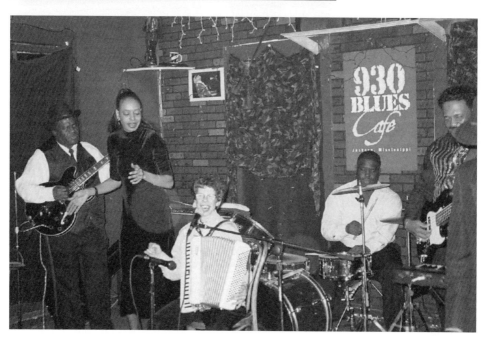

Gloria expands her musical horizons, performing the blues with 930 Blues Club guitarist King Edward, vocalist Jackie Bell, and Ironing Board Sam in Jackson, Mississippi. *Photo courtesy of the Lenhoff family.*

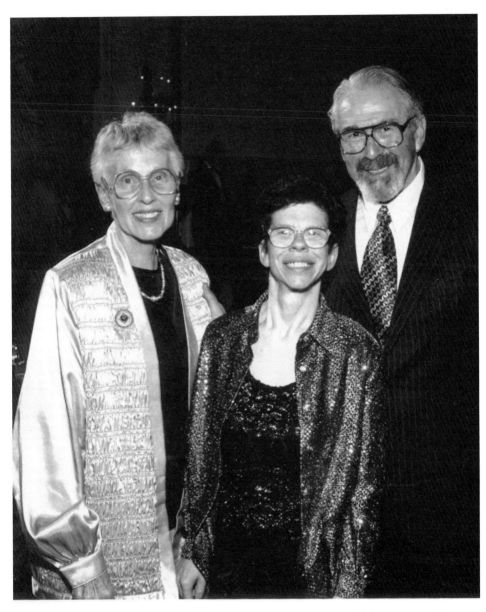

Sylvia, Gloria, and Howard pose after the performance at a Berkshire Hills fund-raiser in Boston. *Photo courtesy of the Lenhoff family.*

{chapter 10}
THE GENES OF
PERSONALITY

The cheers of encouragement and delight that ricocheted through Belvoir Terrace during the Williams camp raised all sorts of interesting, and uncomfortable, questions. It was far out of the range of regular behavior, the unwavering support Williams people offered one another. A person could get up on stage and give the most painful performance imaginable, but still, his Williams friends were wildly supportive and enthusiastic. They seemed to have an uncanny capacity to understand how the person on stage felt, and what would make them feel even better. It seemed, to those who worked at camp, that these were indeed some of the most empathetic and caring people they had come across.

Researchers at the University of Louisville had long heard anecdotes of how very empathetic Williams people were, but they were just that: anecdotes. The scientists wanted facts and measurements. But how do you measure human empathy?

Carolyn B. Mervis and researchers Melissa L. (Thomas) Rowe and Angela M. Becerra started with two groups of four-year-old children. One group had Williams, the other was developing normally. The researchers had two questions: Could children so young display as complex an emotion as empathy? And if so, how did Williams kids compare to regular kids in expressing it?

There were twenty-one kids in the Williams group, fifteen in the regular group. Each child went into a playroom with a researcher, and they played together with toys as a video camera whirred. Researcher Rowe was taken aback by how intensely the Williams kids stared at her.

After a few minutes, Rowe got up and pretended to smack her knee on a table. "Ouch!" she yelled, grabbing her knee and rubbing it for forty seconds, which is a deceptively long time. What happened next startled her: The overwhelming majority of the statements made by Williams children—86 percent—expressed concern, offering to call for help, get a Band-Aid, kiss the boo-boo. Some actually went to the table and pretended to hit their knees, too, saying, "Ow, ow." In striking, and somewhat dismaying, contrast, only 25 percent of the statements made by regular kids expressed concern. The other 75 percent of their utterings were about toys in the room and other things besides Rowe's distress.

Videotapes revealed that, while Rowe was in "pain," 80 percent of the Williams kids focused intensely on her, while only 30 percent of the regular kids did. The regular kids seemed much more centered on themselves, Rowe said; many tried to lure the "injured" researcher back to play with them, rather than offering help or acknowledging her pain. It struck Rowe how little empathy the regular kids seemed to have for others' feelings— and, frankly, it hurt her feelings a bit. The Williams kids, in contrast, almost felt like it was happening to them.

But why? Rowe thinks it relates to two other critical components of the Williams personality profile: overfriendliness and anxiety. Williams people are almost magnetically attracted to people: they love to be around them, to talk to them, to look at them. Perhaps that's partly why they respond so empathetically—they're deeply interested in what is happening with other people. But Rowe also suspects that their own anxieties play a role. Williams people often worry about rejection, and Rowe thinks this fear—and, perhaps, their desire to be liked—is woven into their concern for others. Whatever the reasons, Rowe believes that the root of this personality trait is genetic.

Other researchers were delving into the rich social interactions of Williams people and asking similarly difficult questions. They tried to answer them with experiments that drew on philosophy as well as science.

Most species are wired to respond to the actions of their peers. When the herd erupts into a stampede, the single antelope senses danger and runs, too. But only humans—and, maybe, some primates—can respond to what they believe is the *mental state* of their peers, Salk's Ursula Bellugi and her British colleague Annette Karmiloff-Smith wrote. It's quite a complicated task, requiring a person to make inferences about the contents of another's mind. Did Williams people have "theory of mind"?

Bellugi and Karmiloff-Smith's subjects were eighteen Williams people between ages nine and twenty-three. The experimenter showed a tantalizing packet of M&M's and asked, "What's inside?" The Williams subjects shouted, "M&M's!" But when the experimenter opened the packet, there weren't M&M's inside at all: instead, there were small pencils. After the surge of chocolate-induced disappointment subsided, the experimenter asked what someone who hadn't yet seen inside would think was inside.

This task measured if Williams kids could differentiate between three things: (1) what they knew to be true; (2) what they figured another child would think; and (3) what they predicted another child's response would be, based on what they thought the other thought (rather than what they knew to be true).

While only 20 percent of autistic people scored well on tests like these, Williams people scored phenomenally high: 94 percent of Williams subjects predicted behavior successfully, saying that someone who hadn't yet seen inside the M&Ms bag would think M&Ms were inside. These were easy tasks, which healthy four-year-olds could pass, but they indicated that Williams people could, to a degree at least, climb inside another's mind.

This line of inquiry interested Helen Tager-Flusberg as well. She earned her doctorate in experimental psychology at Harvard University and was a professor at Boston University School of Medicine. She was satisfied that Williams people had theory of mind. She knew how charming and sensitive they could be, and how interested they were in other people. There was something special about their ability to connect; it was one of the things that made Williams syndrome fundamentally different from autism, where people turned radically inward and had little concept of others. But what was really happening with the social perception of Williams people? How did they manage to interpret the behavior of others, to understand their feelings and thoughts? What was the mechanism?

Tager-Flusberg and her colleagues knew that Williams people spent an inordinate amount of time staring at others' faces. They had a hunch this had something to do with their ability to connect. So they decided to see how well Williams people did "reading the windows to the soul."

They formed three groups of adults: thirteen with Williams syndrome; thirteen with Prader-Willi syndrome (a different genetic disorder that results in a similar IQ); and twenty-five regular adults. All were given the "eyes task"—a test based on the idea that there is a "language of the face," that mental states register there for all to see, and that those who understand this concept can identify the contents of another's mind. It's a direct measure of the ability to interpret facial expressions—and a test that high-functioning adults with autism regularly fail.

A long, narrow black-and-white photograph flashed on a screen. There were eyes, and not much else; the image began just above the eyebrows and ended at the bridge of the nose. It was two inches high and five inches wide, a thin strip taken from a larger picture in a popular magazine.

Then two phrases describing polar-opposite emotions were read out loud: "Concerned, unconcerned." "Attraction, repulsion." "Relaxed, worried." "Sad thought, happy thought." "Friendly, hostile." "Flirtatious, not interested." "Calm, anxious." The subject had to say which word described the picture.

Of the regular adults tested, 92 percent passed—that is, got at least seventeen out of twenty-five correct. Of the Williams people, 62 percent passed. Of the Prader-Willi people, only 23 percent passed. As expected, regular adults did significantly better than the Williams adults; but Williams adults performed significantly better than Prader-Willi adults, even though they were matched for age, IQ, and vocabulary. To everyone's surprise, nearly half the Williams people scored as well as regular adults.

The ability to "mentalize," that is, understand the content of another's mind, is relatively intact, but not completely intact, in Williams people, the researchers concluded. The results were more fodder for those who believed in the separate domains of intelligence: It probably meant that the ability to read mental states in people's eyes is a skill that's somewhat independent of general cognitive ability. It might be because the neural systems important in face processing and "mentalizing" are relatively preserved in the Williams brain. It might have something to do with how Williams infants and children spend so much more time staring intensely at people's faces than do regular children. This "attentional difference," aided by their strong interest in people and their outgoing personalities, might let them gather more social information than would otherwise be expected, thus helping them form ideas about the contents of other people's minds.

Tager-Flusberg wanted to know more about the social intelligence of her subjects. Faces provide a great deal of social information, but so do words. She turned her attention to their ability to understand nonliteral language—metaphor, irony, sarcasm. Nonliteral language, she and her colleagues wrote, is at the intersection of language and theory of mind; being able to understand it is a crucial skill for successful social interaction, especially with peers.

Adolescents with Williams were compared to matched groups of adolescents with Prader-Willi syndrome and nonspecific mental retardation. Subjects listened to stories that ended in either a lie or an ironic joke; they were asked to decide which it was, and why.

Despite their social and language strengths, none of the teens with Williams could tell the difference between lies and ironic jokes. For the most part, both lies and ironic jokes were treated as lies, because they did not correspond to reality. The Williams people were significantly more likely to interpret jokes literally than the others, and their errors were similar to those made by younger, normally developing children.

To take the inquiry a step farther, Tager-Flusberg and her colleagues designed what could be called an experiment in social morality. They presented a story, told with pictures, to the Williams subjects: It was about Sally and Mark, two friends who made a date to go to the movies. Sally got all dressed up, went to the theater and waited, but Mark never showed up. In one version of the story, Mark decided that he simply didn't want to go to the movies and stayed home to watch TV. In another version, he tried to take a bus to the theater but the bus broke down. Was Mark's behavior in the first story better than in the second story?

Answering that question required complex thought processes and judgments — understanding the difference between an external force getting in the way of good intentions, and willfully and inconsiderately breaking a date. The Williams people weren't good at it. They couldn't really decide which was worse, Tager-Flusberg said. They couldn't see that there was a difference.

Karmiloff-Smith, Bellugi, and colleagues also tried to measure the higher-order skills of Williams people, this time by testing their understanding of metaphor and sarcasm. Metaphor requires a person to comprehend the links between intended meaning and real meaning; sarcasm requires a person to understand the speaker's attitude, and that what is meant is exactly the opposite of what is said.

Williams people were told a story about a child who was baking a cake and dropped eggs—shell and all—into the batter. One parent says, "Your head is made of wood" (metaphor) while another parent says, "Now that's a clever thing to do" (sarcasm). When the Williams person was asked to explain what the parents meant, only half understood both sarcasm and metaphor. That's a big dip from their performance on simpler tasks, but much better than the overwhelming majority of autistic people. Sarcasm was easier for them to grasp than metaphor.

The conclusion that Bellugi, Karmiloff-Smith, and the others drew was that Williams people might be showing another "islet" of relatively intact ability. Williams children may, with time and experience, develop a social intelligence that they use to understand the world. That's more support for the theory that intelligence isn't an across-the-board affair, and that the adult brain is composed of semi-discrete, at least semi-independent, systems. It also suggests that brain organization is not hard-wired, and that there may be no such thing as "fixed neural architecture." The brain appears to be flexible enough to rewire itself to do what it needs to do, as best as it can.

It is said that everything is better the second time around, and ideas for Williams music camp no. 2 were already whirring. Nancy Goldberg decided everyone would have piano lessons this time. Piano provides instant gratification; the very first stroke of a finger creates a perfect sound. Not so for brass, woodwinds, and stringed instruments. There would also be more music teachers, so everyone could have lessons in drums and voice. There would be more aides, drawn from the ranks of Belvoir's former campers, to help the Williams kids do everything they needed to do. And there would be more campers—they'd increase enrollment to sixty. No one would accuse Nancy Goldberg of being sentimental to her face, but all her planning told a different story—as did the sheer volume of videotape she blazed through during the first camp. There were hours and hours of it. She edited it down to a concise twenty-two minutes, and sent it to the country's half-dozen Williams syndrome clinics. People had to *see* this to believe it.

Howard and Sharon were busy making changes for a bigger, better second camp as well. They designed a new application form to more easily highlight kids' musical interests, put together a packet of extra information for parents who were curious but uncommitted, drew up new guidelines for "camp readiness" to avoid first-time-away-from-home difficulties. They also mounted a major offensive to spread the word about music, and the camp, to other Williams families.

Sharon wrote reports for the association's board, sounding like a lawyer trying to persuade a skeptical jury. "The music and arts camp in Lenox made history: It was not only the first camp created for our Williams Syndrome Association members, but also the nation's first camp to train the musical talents of people with a mental disability. . . ." To illustrate the camp's positive effects, she quoted parents directly:

> This camp has meant hope in the future for our kids. They can do wonders when given a chance. . . . For me, camp has helped to fulfill a need that my child has had in regard to the performing arts, especially music. I have never seen so much enthusiasm and love. . . . This experience was tremendous! I never dreamed it would be so worthwhile . . . we are all coming away from here very enriched by the love for each other and the doors opened for us through music. . . . It was fascinating to see them all together, being real friends. . . . This week gave me a chance to enjoy my son and other WS kids/adults on their level—not the reverse, in which my son is expected to conform to the "regular" world.

The association's board was pleased. To Howard's great surprise, members gave him a hearty round of applause, and Sharon got the OK to write a standing feature in the association newsletter: "Camp Connection," it would be called.

"The Music Camp of 1994 was a first step toward discovering the special abilities of our Williams syndrome children," she wrote. "Since then, many campers have pursued new musical opportunities. . . . Jessica Mavro, 23, auditioned for and was accepted into an opera workshop at Queens College. . . . Carol Burdine, 35, is studying voice with a former Belvoir counselor. . . . Alec Sweazy, 10, has located a Suzuki-trained piano teacher and is proud that already he can play Bach's Minuet in G Major. . . . Anne McGarrah, 46, has acquired a piano and is taking lessons after a lapse of 30 years. . . . John Libera, 14, experienced in piano and saxophone, tried clarinet at camp and now has lessons from a young talent scholarship winner. . . . Gloria Lenhoff, 40, has taken up keyboard. . . . "

And Tori Ackley, ten, was taking the piano and voice lessons that Nancy Goldberg had prescribed for her. That inspired the local school district to assign Tori a music therapist; Kim came over twice a week. When Tori's father Bob came home from work one night, Tori and Kim announced that Tori had written her first song, "Why I Like Snow." The lyrics had young Tori gazing out a window at a fresh field of frosty white, marveling at its beauty, but unsure what she should do next: "Build a snowman? / I really don't know. . . . / Then I heard my mom / call me / in for some / hot tea / that made me warm inside then I went outside / back in the snow / where I can hide / away from here. . . . " Bob choked back tears. To him, it was a metaphor for Tori's life. Looking out the window, seeing the wonders, not knowing what to do next, not being able to fully participate. It's beautiful, he told her.

Howard, in collaboration with researchers Linda Levine and Barbara Sandeen, sent a questionnaire to 388 Williams families trying to learn more about Williams kids and music. More than two hundred were returned. Parents said their Williams children were more interested in listening to music, singing, and dancing than their non-Williams children. The differences in interest were statistically significant.

Sharon and Howard were encouraged. They were fielding phone calls from hesitant, but interested, families. There are three things you need to make music a reality in your child's life, Sharon always said: A watch, car keys, and a wallet. A watch, because it takes the commitment of time. Car keys, because you'll do a lot of driving to find a teacher willing to teach your child by ear. And a wallet, because it does cost money. But the expense and inconvenience are quickly forgotten when a child, frustrated because he can't do simple math, finds himself playing a Bach minuet. It's hard work for everyone. But who can put a price tag on such joy?

Famed author and neurologist Oliver Sacks was intrigued by a study of the brains of professional musicians done by Harvard researchers. The brain, like most of the body, is usually symmetrical. There's a structure called the planum temporale just above the ear canal on each side of the brain, important to auditory processing and language, that's mostly symmetrical as well. But in professional musicians, it isn't symmetrical; it's actually bigger on the left side than it is on the right, the researchers found.

Sacks wrote a letter to the editor of *Science*, suggesting that such asymmetry might have something to do with the exceptional musical abilities seen in people with neurodevelopmental disorders such as autism and Williams syndrome.

Ursula Bellugi, Gregory Hickok, and Wendy Jones fired back a letter. In fact, they had already analyzed the planum temporale in four people with Williams syndrome, and what Sacks was hinting at seemed, indeed, to be the case. They used magnetic resonance images to measure the left and right planum temporale, and found that the asymmetry in Williams brains was similar to the asymmetry in the brains of professional musicians. Three of the four Williams syndrome people actually had greater asymmetry than did the musicians, but less than that seen in musicians with perfect pitch. Another interesting thing: the Williams planum temporales had the same surface area as normal brains, despite the fact that the Williams brains were, on the whole, about 20 percent smaller. They did not, however, do any musical tests on their subjects.

"These preliminary data suggest that disproportionate growth, and perhaps exaggerated asymmetry, occur in . . . individuals with Williams syndrome," they wrote. "However, establishing whether this asymmetry is a source of musical ability will have to await more detailed analyses. Also, the fact that individuals with Williams syndrome typically possess exceptional language abilities relative to other cognitive domains and despite mental retardation introduces the possibility that planum temporale asymmetry is related to linguistic abilities rather than, or as well as, musical abilities."

Sharon was excited by the exchange. Oliver Sacks was an internationally best-selling author. His books—*Awakenings, An Anthropologist on Mars, The Man Who Mistook His Wife for a Hat*—plumbed the deepest, darkest, strangest recesses of the human brain and behavior. She knew that Sacks had met Howard and Gloria at the Salk Institute in San Diego, and she knew that Sacks had been impressed by Gloria's singing. Perhaps he'd like to see more. It would be thrilling to have him as an ambassador to spread the word about music and Williams syndrome. So Sharon scrounged up one of Nancy's camp videotapes and sent a letter to Sacks, inviting him to visit music camp as an observer. She knew better than to hold her breath. She popped the package in the mail and didn't think much more about it.

Camp's enrollment deadline was again approaching, and despite Howard and Sharon's extra efforts, applications were only trickling in. After last year's success, they were sure they could get sixty campers; but they had received fewer than forty applications. Why? Why wasn't their message getting out? Why weren't people listening? They understood that some parents were simply overwhelmed by the medical and educational needs of their kids—when parents are dealing with the anguish of heart surgeries and the struggles of teaching their kids to read, music might seem like a frill. Howard and Sharon wished they could convince people that it wasn't a frill at all, that it was more like a path to fulfillment and success. But they'd have to be happy with smaller victories: Sharon opened one application that dramatically began, "Music is Steven's life." Her heart lightened. They were right. They knew they were right.

Back in California, the young Christian film student Craig Detweiler was getting ready to roll.

He drove from Los Angeles to Costa Mesa to have lunch with Howard, Sylvia, and Gloria, and presented his credentials: divinity school, missionary in Japan teaching English, mentor to inner-city kids. He talked his way into film school at the University of Southern California and was now hooked up with an evangelical production company in Europe—EO Productions International. When he proposed doing a documentary on Gloria, Howard explained that Arlene Alda had beat him to it by about a decade. But there was another fabulous story to be done, Howard told Detweiler: a music camp for Williams people had opened in Massachusetts. It was amazing, Howard promised, unlike anything Detweiler would ever see. And it wasn't just Gloria. There were others with incredible talent as well.

Detweiler was struck by Howard's intensity. Howard came across as the classic stage parent, proud and assertive, someone every aspiring performer could use, disabled or not, Detweiler thought. But there was an urgency behind Howard's unflagging enthusiasm. He saw a man growing older, worrying about what would become of his disabled daughter, and wanting the world to appreciate her gifts the way he did. It moved him. Howard promised Detweiler exclusive access to Gloria and the camp. They signed a contract and Gloria's next movie debut was ready to roll. The piece would play the film festival circuit, then run on European television.

To Sharon's surprise, Oliver Sacks responded to her letter inviting him to camp. He was filming a BBC series called *Mind Travelers*, which focused on neurological mysteries, and would like to visit camp with his film crew. It was a thrilling prospect — except that Howard had already made a commitment to filmmaker Detweiler, granting him exclusive access. But this was Sacks at their doorstep. How could they possibly turn him down?

The *Mind Traveler* series was extensive. Sacks would go to Guam, where people were dying of a disease that combined the worst of Parkinson's and Alzheimer's but was neither one. To Louisiana, where Cajuns were born deaf and went blind later in life, but no one knew why. To Pingelap, a Pacific atoll where one out of every ten people was colorblind. And to Southern California for a convention on autism, a visit with a Williams syndrome family, and a meeting with Williams researcher Ursula Bellugi.

Bellugi introduced Sacks to eight-year-old Heidi Comfort, a cherub with thick glasses and a pageboy haircut who greeted him cheerily at the gate of her Los Angeles home. At first blush, she seemed perfectly normal to Sacks, maybe even a bit advanced; she had the assurance and poise of a sociable adult. "Are you guys ready for a muffin now? OK, who's hungry? Come on," Heidi urged, leading Sacks's weary crew into the kitchen as if she had known them for years.

There, Sacks gave Heidi a little test. He draped napkins over the dish of muffins she was offering him and asked how many were there. "Three," she said quickly. "Three?" Sacks could hardly hide the incredulity in his voice. "Only three?" He removed the napkins and asked her to count them. She stopped at eight, sensed that she wasn't right, and added two more. "Ten!" she proclaimed. Sacks counted them. "Thirteen," he said. She grabbed a muffin and gave it to him with a sweet smile, instinctively compensating for her deficit with her strength: "Here, this is your favorite," she said. "Chocolate!"

Sacks followed the family to a mall, where Heidi headed straight for the calculator aisle, apparently still smarting from her poor mathematical performance. In a whispered aside to the camera, Sacks noted how this might be a way to help cope with her problems. The tiny girl wheeled around on him defiantly. "I don't like what you said," she told him. "I don't like it. It hurts my feelings. Please don't say it. OK? I can do a lot, too."

Sacks was stunned. He was whispering, after all. "She caught every word and put me firmly in my place for hurting her feelings," he said. "I was amazed by the acuteness of her hearing. . . . I had not been prepared for such emotional sensitivity, or such disarming directness." Sacks couldn't imagine what was waiting at the Williams syndrome music camp in Massachusetts.

There was a flurry of negotiations with Detweiler and a deal was struck: If Sacks would agree to be interviewed for Detweiler's documentary, Detweiler would waive his exclusivity rights and share camp with the BBC. Sacks would have to promise not to focus on Gloria, and the two crews would give each other a wide berth.

It was agreed. The message of music, and Williams, would be broadcast far and wide.

{chapter 11}

PITCH PERFECT

The second music camp was far different than it had been the year before. There were still only forty campers, but twenty-five were veterans, and many had been dutifully taking the music lessons that Nancy prescribed for them. There was a higher level of competence and sophistication, and a more serious emphasis on musical exploration. Gloria was branching out into pop and folk music—thanks to the help of Jill Dvore, a classical musician and pop singer in Gloria's new summer home of Crescent City, California—and others were stretching, too. Kids with drumsticks turned the playground into an outdoor rhythm clinic, keeping noisy time on swing sets, seesaws, tree trunks, skinny branches. See how each one sounds different? a teacher said as campers moved from swing to seesaw, pounding and nodding.

The campers loved the cameras, mugging like silent-screen stars ready for their close-ups. "Don't be shy, Mr. Sacks!" they cried when they sensed the scientist's reserve. They, of course, had no reserve at all, and were eager to tell everything they knew.

"I describe Williams syndrome as a very rare genetic disease that not many people have," said Meghan Finn, a singer from California at camp for the first time.

"Williams syndrome can happen at conception, when the egg and sperm meet together and your seventh chromosome is damaged," Anne McGarrah explained.

"Their teeth are not in the right places and they have round noses. See my nose? It's round! It's round!" giggled Alyssa Hanwell.

"If we didn't have it, I don't know what we would be like," said Chris Lawson. "It's not my favorite thing to have, but it's all right."

Chris was belting out "Beautiful Dreamer" in class as the teacher played piano and the camera rolled. Chris, who had never heard the song before, wanted to take a stab at playing it on piano himself.

"It's not so much that they are especially accomplished musicians," Sacks whispered excitedly to the camera as Chris slid onto the piano bench, "but that they respond instinctively to music and musical form." Chris immediately began playing "Beautiful Dreamer," with both hands, chords and melody, slightly slower than the usual pace, improvising on the parts he wasn't sure about. "What strikes me so much is, if he forgets something, he can fill in something plausible, or he can embellish," Sacks said. "He has a clear idea of the musical structure. He has extracted these structures and he can play with them. He knows the rules. There is real musical intelligence here. This is not just a rote repetition."

In a dim practice room, Meghan's head lolled with the rhythm of "The Lion Sleeps Tonight" as the teacher strummed it on guitar. Her eyes were closed, and she harmonized freely on the soaring chorus. Sometimes the harmony worked, sometimes it didn't, but it was a spontaneous eruption that sent her into something that resembled a reverie. Meghan had been two when she started plunking out harmonies on the piano, and soon was making up melodies all her own.

"Music is like soup," Meghan said. "It melts down your throat and it's like, *ahhhhhhhhh*, that's so good!"

Sacks was awed. He told the *Boston Globe* that he hadn't seen that much group enthusiasm for music since attending a Grateful Dead concert. "Just as soon as [music] began, everyone there responded," Sacks said. "They got the rhythm, the beat, exactly. They harmonized. They ad-libbed . . . and suddenly one realized this is, among other things, a highly musical species. . . . They do seem to me a people with an identity of their own."

Sacks, still smarting from Heidi's scolding, began to wonder if the Williams syndrome sensitivity to sound was responsible for their unusual responsiveness to music. "All of them love music," he said. "Many have perfect pitch, and most can pick up a tune with extraordinary ease." He strolled through the nearby forest with Michael, a young man who was transfixed by a symphonic buzzing of bees that Sacks could hardly hear; when what sounded to Sacks like a faint human voice wailed in the distance, Michael growled, "Keep the noise down!" as if it were thunderous. As they continued walking, Michael began a rapid monologue, telling Sacks fantastical stories about bees with queens who are three feet long and weigh three hundred pounds.

On the other side of campus, Detweiler and his crew were also being regaled with stories. A young man giggled uncontrollably into their camera, telling the story of how he loved to take things apart when he was a kid. Once, he found a screwdriver and unscrewed all the screws on a chair. His mother sat on the chair, and it promptly collapsed. He laughed guiltily, gleefully, covering his mouth with his hand, then added, "Of course, I learned how to put things back together." A "ba-bum-bum" could almost be heard in the background.

Detweiler was following Gloria, who was working on a difficult piece that demanded great technical skill: Schubert's "Shepherd on the Rock." Legend has it that it was written for a beautiful diva who'd asked Schubert to compose a brilliant aria that would show off the depths of her emotion and the heights of her octaves. The text, in German, is sung by a lonely shepherd from a perch high atop a mountain. The piece cycles through wonder and sorrow to the hopefulness of a new spring, evoking peaks and ravines with a vocal line that soars and plunges and comes very close to yodeling. It was camp director Nancy Goldberg's idea to see if Gloria could do it. Nancy wanted her to stretch.

Gloria started listening to "Shepherd on the Rock" two weeks before camp began. Nancy was at Gloria's very first rehearsal, expecting a rough run-through, and was surprised when Gloria sang it perfectly. Nancy couldn't imagine many trained singers from Juilliard doing a better job. Laura Goldberg, Nancy's daughter, played violin on the piece. Laura was left wondering just how much of music is intellectual and emotional under-standing, and just how much is opening your mouth and having sound come out. She wasn't sure.

The pianist in that trio was Dalit Warshaw, a new teacher on staff that year, a composer and pianist doing her graduate studies at the Juilliard School. She had been teaching music to regular kids for years, but that did nothing to prepare her for this. It was extremely discombobulating to work with people who were, in one way, mentally retarded, and in another way, so miraculously talented, she'd later write in an article for Juilliard.

One of the most amazing campers that year was Brian Johnson, the guitar- and piano-playing songwriter, who had a deep and innate musicality. He'd hug her so hard he squeezed the breath out of her, beeline to the piano, and become so absorbed in his playing that nothing could distract him. His fingers were bent, his thumbs jutted out at unusual angles, but he still played with grace, improvising songs with well-timed lyrics, catchy hooks, and harmonies that she could imagine hearing on the radio. He played bluesy numbers bemoaning lost love on guitar, and gentler originals like "I'm Nothing without You" on piano. "The train is coming down the trail really fast, and I'm not sure if it's going to really last . . . ," he played for her during one lesson.

That's amazing, Dalit said. When did you write it?

I was singing it to myself during breakfast, he said.

Dalit saw that Brian's musical mind was working differently. The harmonies he chose were unusual: While most basic harmonies are constructed from a root note (say, C) and the notes a third and a fifth above it (E and G), Brian would never play three notes together. Instead, he'd play just two notes, with one hand, usually fourths or thirds. Technically, those were called "second inversion chords," but he was oblivious to that.

Brian was playing rhythm with his left hand and melody with his right, which is common fare in pop; but he was using only his index and ring fingers. Dalit wanted to see if she could make him use more fingers and coax him toward more musical complexity.

Would you like to try something different? she asked, and started playing the third movement of Beethoven's *Tempest* Sonata. It had no regular chords. Instead, the notes of a chord were played one at a time, in rapid succession, by both the left and right hands (technically, an arpeggio). This forced the pianist to stretch his hand the span of an octave and use his pinkie.

Brian was excited. He imitated her right hand using his usual fingering—index and ring—and quickly realized how awkward it was. He understood, without being told, that using his pinkie would be much easier and would allow him to get the arpeggio effect. He watched closely as she played it for him one more time, and then was able to play both hands together entirely on his own. She was amazed how quickly he picked it up, and how intuitively he adapted to the demands of the keyboard.

But of all Dalit's students that summer, none could compare to Alec Sweazy, who was now ten. "Alec is really fascinating," she told Detweiler's camera. "He has this poise, like the piano is under his control. He apparently wasn't taught that. It just happens."

In her opinion, Alec was simply brilliant. He could instantly transpose Dimitri Kabalevsky's "Toccatina"—a childhood piano staple—into different keys. They were working on a Bach piece when Alec got distracted by the honking of a saxophone in a nearby practice room; she decided to do a little experiment. Can you find those sounds on the piano? she asked. There was no hunting and pecking, no noodling around, no hesitation: Alec went straight to the notes he was hearing and struck those keys. They were in the key of D sharp. It was completely obvious to him. Dalit wanted to teach him Bach's Invention in F Major 30 — one of the studies Bach wrote to train his eldest son, a child prodigy. The Inventions look deceptively simple, but they are anything but. Alec tried over and over, his mood growing dark and brooding until he exploded in tears, bitterly declaring, "I'll never get it right!" Dalit knew Alec was a great musician in the making. She didn't see that kind of emotion in any of the other students. Among the teachers, the prevailing wisdom was that whatever musical talent Williams people possessed grew from their ability to imitate. But she didn't buy it. If that was true, how did they explain Alec?

She wanted to know if her students understood the emotional content of music the way she did. She played Chopin's Ballade No. 4 in F Minor, op. 52 — a piece critics have called an exalted, intense, and sublimely powerful work, a crucible for a lifetime's experience, a melody that probes the secrets of the soul and culminates in a coda of bone-crushing technical severity. Dalit played different parts of it for her students, then asked how they felt. They responded instantly. "This is very sad." "Lonely." "Angry." "This is so happy!" They were right every time.

Sometimes, it seemed to Dalit, the Williams people didn't seem to have mental disabilities at all. They were "extremely musical people with brilliant ears who felt every phrase and musical inflection instinctively through the core of their being, without even knowing why," she wrote. The musical instinct, she decided, operates more quickly and more definitively than methodical analysis; it was true for musicians, and it was true for Williams people as well. She started to question the way she had been teaching her regular music students — indeed, questioning the way she was taught. Formal music education was a verbal jungle of terminology and abstractions and written notation that was incomprehensible to Williams people, even though the music itself was crystal clear. Why would something as mysterious as musicality need to be explained in words at all?

A few buildings away, drum teacher K. B. McConnell was discovering much the same thing, in a somewhat discomforting way. He started simple, creating a rhythm pattern by slapping his knees and clapping his hands. Camper Aaron Antolewicz clapped along, keeping the beat with uncanny acuteness. K. B. changed the rhythm abruptly, unnaturally, in a way he never would while making music; Aaron instantly followed along. What was so eerie about it, K. B. said, was that Aaron wasn't looking at his hands, which was the logical place to look, and which was where regular students looked during these exercises. Instead, Aaron looked directly, deeply, and intensely into his eyes. It was a locked, unblinking, awelike stare. McConnell even tried one of the toughest tricks in drumming: keeping a 4/4 beat with his right hand, and a 7/4 beat with the rest of his body. It took professionals years to perfect such limb independence. Aaron picked it up without a struggle. It was awesome—and a tad frustrating.

Watching Williams people make music, "one is awe-stricken and yet also filled with a profound sadness," Dalit Warshaw later wrote. "One wonders why it requires a disability to cause such natural talent, why it takes affliction to cause such beauty. What lies in this one half-chromosome that causes its absence to affect the body and brain in such dramatic ways? One also wonders if the very existence of talent is always induced by genetic fluke, if genius and biological deviation are more linked than we might want to think."

The campers lounged on the mansion's great, emerald lawn in the sparkling laziness of the afternoon and talked, talked, talked. Wouldn't it be great if someday we could all go on the road together and do concerts?

Yeah, sighed Meghan, Chris, Brian, and the others.

Do you ever wonder what life would be like if we didn't have Williams syndrome? they mused.

There's days when I think, 'Gee, I wish I didn't know I had it.' It makes me feel bad that I can't do some of the things that normal people do. But when you come to think about that, what is normal and what is abnormal? a voice in the crowd said.

Do you guys wonder what it's going to be like when you're older, like me? Anne McGarrah asked.

The younger campers nodded. "What are we going to do when we get older? What choices do we have? What is the future going to be like for us?" Meghan asked.

Brian, the guitarist and songwriter, nodded as well. "What jobs can you apply for? What things can you do?" The answers were no different now than they were twenty years ago, when Gloria finished school. Precious little had changed.

At night, after the campers were asleep in their bunk beds, their parents gathered in a small house far across the Belvoir campus and puzzled over the same questions. There were coolers full of beer, wine, and soft drinks; they sipped from plastic cups and tried to find answers. What, indeed, was life going to be like for the Williams kids as they got older? What jobs *could* they apply for? What things *could* they do? Music, of course, Howard said. Gloria had spent years assembling first aid kits for low pay, and though she tolerated it because she loved the chance to socialize, he knew she could do so much more with her music. If only someone would let her. She loved working in the preschool with children, playing her accordion and singing with them, but that was a volunteer job. No pay. A person with a talent should be able to make a living with it, disabled or not. A vision of the future still burned in Howard's mind: a year-round, residential music academy for Williams people, a place that would grant them legitimacy, teach them how to be professional musicians, let them perform for the public and create their own unique community. It would be on a university campus. It would have helpers to take care of the things Williams people couldn't do themselves and it would have housing for parents who wanted to live close to their children. If something like that existed, he wouldn't curse every gray hair and wrinkle. So much uncertainty and angst would be gone. The Williams Syndrome Foundation had been talking with the University of California, Irvine, about creating such a place. UCI was interested, was even willing to provide land, if the foundation would raise the money to build the buildings and run the program. Howard had started assembling an honorary board that would come to include luminaries like Elie Wiesel, Eunice Kennedy Shriver, Oliver Sacks, Colin Powell, Placido Domingo, Itzhak and Toby Perlman, and even former president George H. W. Bush.

Some parents leaned forward as Howard spoke. It was a wonderful thing to think about, to dream about. But could it ever come true?

The odds against it seemed enormous, but people had learned by now not to underestimate Howard's dogged persistence. If you bang your head against a wall long enough and your head doesn't break, the wall falls down.

When camp ended this time, movie cameras caught the hugs that seemed like they would last forever, or at least require crowbars to break up. Meghan's mom felt energized, ready to help her daughter find the path to her future. Wouldn't it be incredible if all of us were a little bit like Williams syndrome children? she thought. "The ability to love, to care about each other, to treat one another with compassion. . . . I think there are some messages here," she said.

Detweiler's film took its title from something Sacks said: *Williams Syndrome: A Highly Musical Species*. It did well on the festival circuit, winning a CINE Golden Eagle for excellence in documentary video production and a Crystal Heart for best full-length documentary at the Heartland Film Festival, and was well received when it aired in 1996 in Europe. Detweiler's film showed Williams syndrome as Howard wanted the world to see it, but he was frustrated when American stations declined to pick it up for broadcast.

Sacks's documentary did air on American public television stations. It was called "Don't Be Shy, Mr. Sacks!" after the advice campers gave him at Belvoir Terrace. It displayed their musical acuity, and Sacks's own wonder, in what seemed to be overwhelming anecdotal evidence.

"I think there is no simple neurological basis for the appreciation of music and musical capacity," Sacks concludes in his documentary. "Many different systems of the brain are involved. Some have to do with the recognition of pitch, probably some with rhythm. As far as I can see, all of these systems seem to be heightened with Williams syndrome. . . . It's as if the brain has been stimulated to grow in some ways, and prevented from growing in others. A strange, lop-sided brain, which sort of makes it impossible to use simple terms like 'able' and 'disabled.'"

That was truly music to Howard's ears.

As doggedly as Howard was pursuing the music angle of Williams syndrome, Colleen Morris was pursuing the genetics. "Williams syndrome is very interesting, not just from the standpoint of it can cause mental retardation and it has these heart problems, but also it has a very unique personality associated with it," geneticist Morris told a journalist. "A lot of people are interested in that because there's a question: could one of these genes actually be involved in human personality? That's a very interesting question."

Morris's discovery that the elastin gene was missing from chromosome 7 in Williams people raised more questions in her mind than it answered. She teamed up again with Mark Keating, the University of Utah molecular geneticist who had worked with her to unravel the elastin mystery; and with Carolyn Mervis, a cognitive psychologist at Emory University in Atlanta. What about those other genes Williams people were missing—some twenty of them? What was the link between missing strands of DNA and the specific attributes of Williams syndrome? They wanted to unravel the mystery. But how to proceed?

When they looked at Williams people they saw great variation in their medical symptoms, in the level of their friendliness, in their ability to tell dramatic stories. But one thing never seemed to vary: how terrible they were at visual-spatial tasks. They simply could not think in three dimensions. They couldn't construct pictures in their heads the way other people could. When Oliver Sacks asked Heidi to assemble four cubes in a simple pattern—black, white, white, black—she was utterly unable to reproduce the original, even though it was right in front of her. When Ursula Bellugi asked a child to draw a bicycle, the results were very nearly incomprehensible: one wheel floating lonely here, another isolated far over there, the chain hovering unattached to anything else, while pedals and seat and rider drifted freely in space. Williams people were notoriously unable to follow directions from point A to point B and got lost in shopping malls they had visited a hundred times.

The elastin gene, they knew, could not be responsible for this. There is virtually no elastin in the brain. But Morris and her colleagues had a theory. Perhaps each aspect of Williams syndrome—personality, spatial problems, etc.—was caused by problems with genes nestled close to the elastin gene. People who lost just the elastin gene might get the heart defect. Those who lost two genes might get the heart defect and the visual-spatial thinking problems. Those losing three might have heart and visual-thinking problems as well as the loquacious personality.

Their path seemed clear: the visual-spatial gene was the one they would go after next.

Morris and her colleagues zeroed in on two families. Both were plagued by the heart problems arising from the missing elastin gene, but none had Williams syndrome and all were of normal intelligence. The average IQ was about one hundred, and while many did not finish high school, they held jobs and lived independent lives. But they had great difficulty doing things that involved visual and spatial reasoning. They avoided hobbies like building model ships or airplanes. They steered clear of jobs involving blueprints and drawings and assembling furniture. And, like Williams people, they had trouble reproducing simple block designs when the researchers tested them.

The researchers examined the DNA of twenty-five of these people. Thirteen were missing the elastin gene, as well as the gene right next to it. Was this a visual-spatial gene? Through months of work, they figured out that the new missing gene instructed cells to produce an enzyme called LIM kinase-1. This enzyme is vital in newly forming brain cells, and seems to be important for early development. It's possible that someone with only one copy of LIM kinase-1 could have a defect in the part of the brain that processes visual and spatial information, they said.

In a soon to be controversial paper published in the journal *Cell* on July 12, 1996, Morris and her colleagues concluded that the deletion of the LIM kinase-1 gene caused impaired cognitive development. Such a claim had never been made before. Physical characteristics had been linked to specific genes, but never something as abstract and complex as thinking. It was touted as a scientific breakthrough.

"Our study showed that these people were missing one copy of LIM kinase, which indicates that LIM kinase is involved in normal cognition," Keating said in an interview.

There were stories in the *New York Times* and on National Public Radio. "Scientists have found a gene that seems to underlie a higher form of human thinking—the ability to take things apart mentally, like pieces of an imaginary puzzle, and to reassemble the parts into a whole," the *New York Times* wrote. Ursula Bellugi said the finding opened the possibility that scientists might find other genes involved in behaviors like language, musical talent, and abstract problem solving.

Keating explained it to the *Times* this way: While the brain is taking shape before and after birth, it forms complex networks for complex jobs like vision, hearing, and movement. No one yet knows how these networks evolve, or how they are shaped by experience, or which genes switch on and off to guide their development.

But it's clear that genes that switch on and off exist. If one is bad, it could cause a whole circuit to form incorrectly, which could result in problems with thinking. A single gene will not give rise to a complex cognitive pathway, Keating told the *Times*, but a mutation in a gene that helps construct or regulate that pathway could disrupt the entire system.

Howard and other scientists had great respect for Morris and Keating, but they had trouble with their conclusion. It just didn't make sense to them that something as complicated as visual thinking could hang so heavily on a single gene. Other skeptical researchers would soon prove them right: they found three more people who were missing the LIM kinase-1 gene, gave them the same visual-spatial tests that Morris and Keating gave to their subjects, and found that these folks did just fine. They had no problems with visual-spatial processing.

Morris, for her part, still believes that LIM kinase-1 is among several genes that contribute to visual-spatial processing. Somehow, the loss of it interrupts, or scrambles, the neurological pathway, she has said. How? That remains a mystery. A mystery that a condition like Williams syndrome may someday help solve.

Howard was annoyed that researchers had still failed to do the obvious: investigate possible links between music and Williams syndrome. The success of the second music camp made him more certain than ever that a link existed. The researchers, in turn, were also annoyed that Howard kept pestering them, and at one professional meeting, one burst out, "Lenhoff, you're a scientist. Why don't you do it?"

Howard specialized in biochemistry and enzymes, not behavior and cognition. He had what some might see as a conflict—a personal interest in the topic, and a deep and passionate interest in the outcome. But Howard's greatest interest was in discovering the truth. He was tired of waiting for someone else to do it. If he had to, he would investigate the possibilities himself.

But how? How does one measure musical ability? And what, exactly, does one measure? He recalled the one refrain he heard so often from parents of Williams children, and again from the teachers at camp: so-and-so has perfect pitch.

Perfect, absolute pitch. The ability to hear a single, solitary note, and know that it is a G, or an A, or a B-flat, and to be able to produce that pitch on command. Most trained musicians have relative pitch—that is, they can only make sense of notes in relation to other notes. Only a tiny fraction of people has absolute pitch: just one of every ten thousand people, studies of non-Asian populations had shown. Those who have it said they hear notes the way others see colors: just as you see grass and simply know it's green, they hear a note and simply know it's an A-sharp. There's no conscious thought involved. Absolute pitch is an astonishing ability, and a good, solid measure of innate musicality, Howard thought. Other scientists had measured absolute pitch before, so there was a road map on how to do it. Now, Howard would just have to figure out how to do it with Williams people.

Howard started searching for funding. He explained his ideas to Joseph Young, head of the National Science Foundation's Division of Cognitive Sciences. Young was intrigued, but Howard was considered "high risk"—a scientist reaching beyond his area of expertise. Howard countered that he had changed research fields before, going from biochemistry to marine and invertebrate biology, becoming an expert in small molecules controlling the feeding behaviors of the little hydra and marine sea anemones and dangerous stinging Portuguese men-of-war. He was, first and last, a man of science.

The NSF has a mechanism for awarding grants for such "high-risk" research. Young said he'd consider awarding such a grant to Howard only if he joined forces with an established behavioral scientist.

Howard's search began at UCI. Just across campus was Gregory Hickok, a young cognitive scientist who had worked with Bellugi on studies of language and the brain. Hickok's goal was to understand the neural organization of language. Hickok's lab was using functional imaging, electromagnetic recording, the study of language breakdown in disease states, and a variety of methods to better understand the neuroscience of language. Hickok agreed to help Howard.

There was a young research associate in Hickok's lab named Olegario Perales. Ole had recently earned his undergraduate degree and was trying to figure out whether to go to graduate school or medical school. In the interim, he worked in Hickok's neuroscience lab, as well as with another UCI researcher investigating how hearing works. Ole had studied music. Classical guitar. He wanted to fuse his interest in music with his curiosity about cognition and the brain.

Like a scientific matchmaker, Hickok introduced Howard to Ole. Ole seemed like a serious, soft-spoken, studious young man, and he thought Howard's line of inquiry could fuse areas of interest for him. Ole agreed to sign on.

There were many details to figure out. Their first thought was to do a large and definitive experiment involving four groups: Williams people with no musical training; Williams people with musical training; regular people with no musical training; and regular people with musical training. Everyone would get the same tests, which would allow the scientists to reach definitive conclusions about absolute pitch in the different populations.

But such a comprehensive approach had one big problem. It

meant that someone—the researchers?—would have to teach all the nonmusicians, Williams and regular, the names of the notes. The subjects had to know that, or a foolproof measure of perfect pitch was impossible. Ole thought of it this way: someone might be able to *use* a pen, but unless they spoke English, they wouldn't be able to *call* it a pen. The researchers needed to find people who spoke the language of music whether they were musicians or not.

They settled on a smaller vision. They would test only Williams people who already knew the names of the notes. They'd compare them to three control groups of university graduates: one that had little musical training, another with a great deal of musical training, and another with advanced degrees in music. Howard knew the talent in the Williams world intimately and went to work. Gloria could tell a G from a D, though she wasn't used to assigning names to the tones. The young pianist Alec Sweazy knew them as do, re, mi. There were others as well, for a total of five. All were strongly musical. All had attended Williams camp for years. But did they have absolute pitch?

Howard, Ole, and Hickok agreed on a simple way to test. The experimenter—it would be Ole—would strike a note on the piano. The subject would name the note, sometimes sing it, and then they'd quickly move on to the next trial. Ole was warned about how eager to please Williams people are; he must keep his poker face intact and give no smile, no nod, no indication of whether the answer was right or wrong.

Ole packed his bag and hit the road. He mostly stayed at the homes of the families, sleeping in guest rooms or on sofas, eating meals with them, and testing the subjects for hours each day. He used a Sony Walkman Professional WM-D3 to record the sessions.

His first subject was Gloria. She was forty-two when she learned to name the notes, at Howard's request; something most adults would find nearly impossible to do. Ole struck an A on the keyboard of the living room piano; "A," Gloria said, then searched his face for a sign that she was right. He struck an F;

Gloria said "F." He struck a B; Gloria said "B." He played dyads—two notes at the same time, like C and G—and she named them both. He played triads—three notes at the same— and she named those as well. It went on and on like that, with Gloria getting virtually every answer right.

Then Ole gave her a much more difficult test. He asked her to sing a simple song like "Happy Birthday" in the key of C major, substituting notes for words. That meant "Happy birthday to you" became "C, C, D, C, F, E," and so on. He started in C because it's the simplest key, devoid of sharp and flat notes. Then he said, "Please change the key to G." Gloria obliged. Ole was astonished.

In Minnesota, he tested Alec Sweazy, the lanky kid with the adorable mop of blond hair. Alec was in regular classes at school, in the right grade level for his age, and was clearly the highest-functioning Williams person Ole had met. When Alec sat down at the piano, Ole was nothing less than startled: he played very difficult, very long Rachmaninoff pieces, entirely by ear, entirely from memory. Ole asked Alec to sing the melody of one of the Rachmaninoff pieces and to tell Ole the notes; Alec did it with ease. Ole asked Alec to change the key and to tell Ole the notes again; again, Alec transposed with ease. Ole couldn't believe it. What on earth was happening? It was almost like Alec could see the music in his head. Many professional musicians couldn't do what Alec and Gloria were doing, he thought to himself. Professionals might hear a piece of music, figure out the relationship between the notes and the key, but to tell you right off the bat which notes they were hearing was a rare skill indeed. He wished he could do that; he imagined being able to listen to a song on the radio and just pick up his guitar and play it, rather than sitting there, plunking away, figuring everything out. He tried to damp down pangs of jealousy. How could it be that the same people who had this incredible ability froze with incomprehension when asked simple questions about "more" and "less"— concepts that small children usually understood?

Back home, Ole, Howard, and Hickok crunched data. The Williams people completed nearly 1,100 trials, and correctly identified notes 97 percent of the time. When identifying each note in a dyad or triad, they were right 98 percent of the time. The normal control group averaged only 18 percent correct.

Clearly something was different in the Williams people's ability to hear and process sound. Whatever was happening, it allowed them to develop musical abilities when it seemed that they just shouldn't be able to.

Williams syndrome had come to the attention of producers at *60 Minutes*, the most successful broadcast news magazine in TV history. They would do their own take on the story.

In Howard's constant campaign to get media exposure for Williams and music, this was something like the Holy Grail. As far as mass media goes, it doesn't get much bigger than *60 Minutes*. It had been TV's top-rated show five times and had been in the top ten for twenty-three consecutive years. Its fourteen million viewers dwarfed the million-plus circulations of the *New York Times* and the *Los Angeles Times*. This was the audience, it seemed, Howard had been working toward all these years.

A *60 Minutes* crew would be at the 1996 Belvoir Terrace music camp to do a piece on Williams syndrome. Veteran anchor Morley Safer would catch up with campers later and interview them himself.

Association director Terry Monkaba—who had been on the front lines of parental frustration over Howard and music—had bought her crimson-haired son Ben a drum set. He had severe attention difficulties, but was doing remarkably well at concentrating during his drum lessons. That Ben, now twelve, could hold drumsticks and keep a steady beat when he didn't have the motor control to tie his shoes or button his shirts seemed terribly incongruous. Ben had suffered terrible health crises as a child, including four heart surgeries, but he radiated that signature Williams warmth and friendliness, and had an amazing memory for faces. So when the *60 Minutes* crew walked into the theater, Ben's face lit up. "Morley? Morley Safer?" Ben asked, his smile cracking wide.

"Yes, himself," Safer said. Ben grabbed Safer's hand and pumped it enthusiastically, almost loath to let go.

"How are you?!" Ben asked, and he really wanted to know.

Whatever professional skepticism Safer might have had didn't stand a chance with this crowd. Safer was swept up on a wave of Williams hospitality as Gloria, Meghan, and a half-dozen others crowded around to introduce themselves, shake hands, and occasionally hug him. Then they all had a sit-down chat in front of the cameras. "Tell me, how important is music to any of you?" Safer asked. Meghan had perfected her answer to this question and didn't need a second to think: "Music is a huge part of my life," she said. "To me, music is like soup: music comes down your throat and feels so warm. So music is like soup. It tastes good." Safer was obviously charmed; Howard noted that Meghan had used the same lines many times before, as Williams people tend to do. They find out what works and they stick with it, and can give the impression that they are so much more intelligent and savvy than they really are.

"Gloria, how many languages can you sing in?" Safer asked.

Gloria closed her eyes like a contented cat and said, "Twenty-five languages."

"Twenty-five?"

"Yes, absolutely," she said.

"Apart from the obvious ones . . ."

"I could sing in Macedonian, Korean, Bulgarian, Yiddish, you name it," Gloria said.

Safer did his own on-screen test of their very sensitive hearing — the trait that had gotten Oliver Sacks into such trouble with Heidi — by turning away from them and whispering into his hand. The microphone picked up a faint mumble, but immediately Meghan blurted out *"What time is it!"* and they all fell to boisterous laughter.

"Are you really happy most of the time?" Safer asked, and there was a chorus of yeses.

"We can't help it," the children said. Howard had a feeling they said what they thought Safer wanted to hear, eager as always to please.

When Sharon was guiding the *60 Minutes* crew through music camp, she pointed out a visitor who hadn't had any contact with other Williams people before, thinking they might find his experience fresh and interesting. He stole the show: Michael Williams had the rare combination of being musically accomplished *and* extremely charming and talkative. Michael also had drama: His face was long and thin, his dark hair was parted on the side and slicked back, his misshapen teeth were almost always on display in a smile. He strolled the paths of Belvoir Terrace singing the lyrics "Please release me, let me go, for I don't love you anymore" under his breath, and the camera was glued to him.

Michael was in his late thirties, and his family had gotten the diagnosis of Williams syndrome only recently. Visiting camp was a revelation for him, much as the first Williams picnic had been for Howard and Gloria a decade earlier.

"Was that a terrific feeling to know that, somehow you really weren't an oddball anymore?" Safer asked as Michael rocked to and fro at the keyboard of a black grand piano.

"Oh, yeah," Michael said. "Somehow I felt that I fit in."

Michael's parents had made sure all their children took piano lessons—except Michael. They couldn't imagine he could do it. But after the other kids finished their lessons and ran out to play, Michael slid onto the bench and noodled around, plunking keys for hours. His parents were shocked when, one day, he played "What Now, My Love," a song recorded by Herb Alpert and the Tijuana Brass. Now he was playing spirited, sprightly pieces with ragtime sensibility and dance hall abandon.

Michael cocked his head to the side and grinned. "Can I play you a song?" he asked Safer, launching into a high-spirited rag that began, "Listen here, boys, I'm telling you now . . ." and ended with an enormous grin and, "I'm a *60 Minutes* Maaaaaaaaaaaaan!" Safer grinned back, clearly charmed.

"Tick, tick, tick, tick, tick, tick, tick," Safer said. "That was great, Michael. Thank you."

When the segment aired in 1997 and 1998, it was like the genie had finally popped out of the bottle. Safer, seated before a giant blow-up of the human brain, intoned in a commanding tenor, "The brain. That most complex of all organs, the one that defines us in more ways than we can even think about. There are forty thousand genes in the brain, and if only a few of those are missing, the result can be devastating—and fascinating. For example, a condition called Williams syndrome, a birth defect in which about twenty of those genes are missing. Scientists believe that by studying people with Williams, they can start to solve some of the mysteries of the human mind.

"Most people with Williams syndrome have an unusual appearance and are generally considered retarded," Safer continued. "But what interests scientists is not just what they can't do but what they *can* do, and what their disabilities and talents may reveal about the rest of us."

The piece did what Howard had long hoped for: highlight the link between music and Williams in a manner that seemed irrefutable, for an audience of millions.

The same summer the *60 Minutes* crew showed up, Ursula Bellugi, the Salk researcher Howard had hounded for so long and who had made such fascinating observations about Williams and language, agreed to visit camp. She, too, would look further into the mysterious musicality of Williams people, even though she knew it would be extremely difficult to measure. Because it wasn't her area of expertise, she would bring along a researcher named Daniel Levitin, a cognitive psychologist who had just earned his doctorate from the University of Oregon, who also happened to be an experienced sound engineer, record producer, and bass player. If anyone could lend insight, he could.

{*chapter 12*}
SING OF
RICE KRISPIES

"I have Williams syndrome!" Meghan Finn roared, whipping the microphone cord around like a seasoned lounge singer. "I was born with it on September 2, 1976. I don't know if any of you have birthdays in September, but we Virgos rock!"

The audience, about two dozen senior citizens who had not rocked for quite some time, laughed. They lived near Belvoir Terrace and had come to love these concerts given each year in conjunction with the Williams music camp. "Williams syndrome doesn't make me stupid," Meghan told them. "I feel Williams syndrome has given me challenges and a lot of gifts, more gifts than I can ever imagine in my whole life. I can't stand loud noises, but I like to sing. I have flat feet, but I like to be with people. I have a definite explosive personality! Just remember us by our talents. We don't have stupidity. We just have love." Then Meghan launched into one of her trademark numbers, a vampy version of "The Glory of Love" that had her crisscrossing the stage, tossing her head back, and thrusting her arms toward heaven like a Las Vegas showgirl. She was, in technical terms, a ham's ham.

Meghan was high functioning enough to study music at college, live in a dorm, and feel the pain of struggling to find her place in the world. Her classmates were so nice to her in class, but they never called after class was over, never asked her to lunch, never invited her to the movies. Meghan didn't quite fit in; she was smart and sensitive enough to know she didn't fit in. It broke her parents' hearts. But on stage, in the spotlight, the friendly girl with few friends suddenly became the belle of the ball. Few at Belvoir had the stage presence of Meghan, and the scientists would soon see that for themselves.

Howard and the other parents were thrilled that Ursula Bellugi, one of the world's preeminent Williams researchers, wanted to visit Belvoir with scientist and musician Daniel Levitin. But when the scientists asked about doing some explorative research while there, brows furrowed. There was the pledge that Howard, Sharon, and Nancy had made years ago: camp was for kids to have fun and enjoy music, not to be poked or prodded or investigated by scientists. It was their chance, for once, to not be different. Scientists could come a day early or stay a day later if they wanted to do something formal, but research during camp itself was out of the question.

Could they make an exception? Sharon, Howard, and Nancy grappled and debated, then reached what they considered to be an acceptable compromise: the scientists could stay as long as they liked and *observe*. Quietly. Unobtrusively. Like flies on the wall. They were to leave the kids alone and let them enjoy themselves; if they brainstormed up a formal study to do in the future, that could be discussed later. Bellugi and Levitin agreed.

Levitin was an unusual scientist, and he cut quite a contrast to the matriarchal Bellugi. He had a mop of dark hair, a faint resemblance to Bob Dylan, and the loose carriage of a rock 'n' roller who'd played one beer bar too many. The expression on his face suggested he was always faintly amused: Levitin had once worked as a stand-up comic and was proud of winning the National Lampoon Standup Comedy Competition regional finals in 1989.

He came to science from the record business. Levitin was,

most recently, president of artists and repertoire for 415/Columbia Records in San Francisco, but had also worked as a session musician, recording engineer, and live sound engineer, and had produced and consulted on more than thirty rock and pop records, including work by Joni Mitchell, Steely Dan, Stevie Wonder, and the Carpenters. He had performed live with Mel Tormé, Nancy Wilson, and the Steve Miller Band. He had built custom guitar amplifiers for Blue Oyster Cult, Joe Satriani, and Chris Isaak. Sound had fascinated him since he was a small boy: He got his first tape recorder at age four, and was soon taping his parents' private conversations, much to their dismay. He took up saxophone and bass guitar, made demo tapes with his buddies, and went to MIT, only to leave shortly after his stereo caught fire in the dorm while listening to *Abbey Road* (really, really loud). He transferred to Stanford University to study music and psychology but dropped out, became the bass player for a San Francisco punk band called Judy Garland (which played originals like "Rats on High," about a junkie flopping in a vermin-infested basement), and shared the stage with some big names, including Sonic Youth. Judy Garland split up over creative differences, but to this day Levitin believes they could have been as big as rockers the Smithereens if they had only stayed together.

While he was still producing records, Levitin started sitting in on lectures at Stanford. Why was some music successful while other music wasn't? Why was some music considered "good" while other music wasn't? It all seemed wound up with how the brain processes music, and neuropsychology came closest to answering his questions. He returned to Stanford for his BA and went on to get a doctorate in psychology from the University of Oregon. When Bellugi asked her colleagues if they knew of anyone who could study music scientifically, she was sent to Levitin. Within a week, he was meeting with Bellugi and hearing of Belvoir Terrace.

Levitin was skeptical whether they would find anything of

scientific value at Belvoir Terrace. He knew there were always fascinating cases of individuals—Sacks's *Man Who Mistook His Wife for a Hat*, for instance—but there was no "mistook his wife for a hat" syndrome. There weren't people everywhere mistaking their wives for hats. These were one-of-a-kind cases, idiosyncratic affairs that happened once and were never repeated. That was probably what was happening at Belvoir Terrace, Levitin felt. The idea that people with profound developmental disabilities could still be musical seemed, to him, most unlikely. Maybe there were one or two, but, for him, one or two was not enough. He needed to see many different examples before he could draw any conclusions. When he expressed his doubts to Bellugi, she said, Just give me one week. They would think of themselves as anthropologists—open-minded, without assumptions, stepping into a new situation, and simply observing. He agreed, and soon they were on their way to Massachusetts.

As Levitin strolled Belvoir's hilly campus, the first thing that struck him was how very well behaved the Williams kids were. He had been a counselor at a summer camp with the same kind of gravel drive Belvoir had, and had yelled himself hoarse trying to stop kids from hurling rocks at one another. But these kids couldn't care less about the rocks on the drive. They weren't throwing things at one another, they weren't pulling hair, they weren't shoving. No roughhousing at all. It seemed different than most gatherings of kids he was familiar with.

Levitin was armed with a video camera and a Sony digital audio recorder, and he and Bellugi roamed campus from early in the morning until long after the parents concluded their nightly sessions. They heard about the kid who had a passion for vacuum cleaners and owned eighteen of them. About the kid who was so fascinated with lawn mowers that he begged his parents for one and now mowed all the lawns in the neighborhood. About the kid who could identify cars solely by the sound of their motors. These kids couldn't turn off sounds that other people tended to ignore;

Levitin and Bellugi came to think of this as their "soundscape sensitivity."

As they visited classes and watched the Williams kids sing, dance, and play piano, guitar, and drums, it became obvious that there was a great range in their musical abilities. Just as there'd be in any population. But one thing did not seem to vary at all: their incredibly high degree of engagement with music. Levitin and Bellugi watched as kids made their way from one class to another, from dining hall to dorm room, singing to themselves or in groups, playing instruments as they walked. They weren't showing off or being self-consciously *musical*, as regular music camp kids might; they were simply having a blast. It reminded Levitin of when he saw Ray Charles for the first time, the unabashed way Charles rocked back and forth, joyfully possessed with the music. Completely uninhibited. You just didn't find that at most gatherings of school-age musicians.

Music wasn't just a deep part of their lives, but an ubiquitous, all-pervasive, omnipresent one, Levitin and Bellugi agreed. When one camper came upon another making music, no matter how informally, the newcomer either joined in immediately or began swaying appreciatively in time, and was always, always welcomed. It wasn't simply loving music, Levitin felt; it was a "consuming involvement." In all his years as a professional musician, he rarely encountered this type of total immersion and natural musical connectedness—even though it was the goal of every professional musician he had ever known. Without effort, the Williams musicians were in what psychologists call "flow"—a state of deep enjoyment and concentration that allows absolute and utter absorption.

At the very end of the day, Levitin and Bellugi would meet, trying to figure out what it all meant and what was there to study. At first, it seemed logical to plan a test for absolute pitch: it showed up often in people with autism and other developmental disorders. But Howard was already working on that. The more they listened, the more drawn they were to pinning down what the Williams parents meant when they called their children "musical." They wanted to quantify these claims of musicality and divide them into component pieces—rhythm, melody, memory for music, performance, listening skills. They intended to draw up a long-term plan for their research, but it struck them that they didn't have to wait and design a big experiment to test rhythm; they could do it right then and there, quietly, unobtrusively.

Much work had been done on the musical abilities of mentally disabled people, and Levitin read many of the same studies that Canadian researcher Audrey Don had read years before. The studies found that savants excelled at musical tasks involving melody and harmony, but had a much harder time with rhythm. Tests done on people with Down syndrome—who, much like Williams people, showed great responsiveness to music—found that they had delayed rhythmic responses and couldn't keep a beat. It seemed reasonable to suppose that Williams people might have trouble keeping a beat as well.

Would you like to play a rhythm game? Levitin would ask a camper, artfully bending the no-research-during-camp rule. The answer was often an enthusiastic yes. The two would sit down at the picnic tables overlooking the mansion's expansive lawn. I'm going to clap a rhythm, he told the child. When I'm done, I'd like you to copy it and clap it back to me. Then Levitin began to clap. At first, the patterns were simple, including the classic "shave-and-a-haircut," minus "two bits." Then they progressed to more and more difficult patterns, like syncopated "swing time," where the rhythm doesn't fall on accented beats. There were twenty patterns in all, based on those used in the Gordon Musical Aptitude Profile.

One of the first things Levitin noticed was how all the campers looked him dead in the eye, rather than watching his hands, as one might expect. It was the same thing that had intrigued the drum teacher years earlier. Levitin would pick a rhythm: *Clap, clap, clap-clap, clap*, and he was surprised to find the Williams kids clapping back immediately, on the next beat, without pausing, as if their response was an extension of the original. Levitin tried to figure out why that would be: perhaps it was because he held his hands together in the closed position after he finished clapping the last beat, and the Williams kids took that as their cue to begin. But to come in immediately, on the beat? That was something else, something he had not been expecting.

As the trials got more difficult, the Williams kids were able to track changes in the rhythmic pulse, from swing time to straight eighths to triplets to sixteenths. Sometimes he started the next trial immediately after the children finished their claps, creating the vibe of a jazz jam session of "trading ones," a technical term used to describe musicians who alternate playing a musical phrase.

These people had poor coordination. They had fingers that tended to act in unison rather than independently. Some found it difficult to get food from plate to mouth. But still they managed to play clarinets, pianos, drums, guitars, and accordions, which required a much finer degree of control and coordination than they seemed to possess. The playing wasn't technically perfect, but he couldn't help but feel that they more than compensated for that with their musicality.

Like so many visitors before him, Levitin was captivated by Brian Johnson, the piano- and guitar-playing singer whose parents followed him around with a tape recorder to catch the original songs that constantly spilled from him. Levitin and Brian sat in a practice room. Levitin asked Brian if he had a favorite breakfast cereal. "Rice Krispies!" Brian said. Levitin asked if Brian could write a song about Rice Krispies. Sure, Brian said, and immediately started riffing on the piano:

> Rice Krispies sound all right
> Until somebody came along, and it was dark at night

> And then all of a sudden I heard them say
> "You sure do like Rice Krispies"
> 'Cause you finally know that you've got to eat
> I said, "Well yeah, I do"
> But then somebody told me
> That they were gonna steal them from me
> 'Cause I didn't know what to do with it
> Then I put some milk in the bowl
> And I said, "That's not gonna do it"
> So whenever you're eating Rice Krispies
> Be sure you put some milk in it
> And then just enjoy yourself
> And then just eat it all up
> And then you are feeling mighty well

Levitin was shocked and delighted. A spontaneous song from someone who, allegedly, had profound disabilities. Brian's voice was natural, had great presence, and was characterized by a complete lack of inhibition, even as he played nearly all of his piano chords in "root" position—that is, with nearly identical fingerings. That could be a result of the poor muscle coordination typical of Williams, Levitin thought.

Levitin wondered if this song was simply a knock-off of something Brian had written before, so he asked Brian to play more of his original work. There was quite a repertoire, but the Rice Krispies song had a distinct compositional style and a marked melodic originality.

Fascinated, Levitin asked Brian if he had a favorite animal. My dog, Brian said, and on the spot, launched into another new song:

> A dog starts to bark
> A dog starts to get mean
> A dog starts to sing

And then she starts to scream
The dog starts to sigh
Then the dog starts to cry
Then the dog starts to growl
Then I start tonight. . . .
But then I sit down to watch TV
And then I turn out the light
And I say, "That dog is staying out tonight." . . .
But then one day the police came along
And tried to take my dog away
But then I said, "Hmm"
That sure is a price to pay
But then she came back
And then I started to go slack
Because then she finally started to growl at me. . . .

Structurally it was sophisticated, Levitin felt. Brian made clever rhymes. He used assonance, a rhyme that repeats similar vowel sounds, as in the phrase "tilting at windmills." His first two verses shared a parallel structure (a dog/the dog). The fourth lines switched to pronouns (she/I). The narrator shifted viewpoint from the third person to the first person—something Brian also did in the Rice Krispies song—which, Levitin hypothesized, was probably a "compositional predisposition."

Brian's songs had standard structural elements, like repeating and developing motifs, but both lacked a traditional chorus. Levitin didn't think that was so unusual; accomplished songwriters often didn't form a chorus so early in the songwriting process. At this first-blush stage, they were still playing with word sounds and with melodic variations. The sound of words was critical in this early phase, even if the words didn't make sense: Paul McCartney's original lyric for "Yesterday" was "scrambled eggs" (each had three syllables), and Paul Simon's original lyric for "Kodachrome" was "goin' home." If you saw Paul Simon's first drafts, Levitin said, the songs might seem very much like Brian's. In Levitin's opinion, the quirks and imperfections in Brian's lyrics were typical first attempts at creating a song.

There was only one explanation for what he saw at Belvoir: Whatever it is in the brain that's required for music making is, to some degree, separate. There was obviously functional independence between processing circuits. The way scientists had long thought about brain architecture seemed to be wrong.

If you had told Kay Bernon a few years ago that her son Charles could be absolutely and utterly absorbed in anything for more than five minutes, she would have laughed. Kay was the philanthropist who had been so filled with hope when she saw Gloria sing at the 1990 Williams Syndrome Association convention. She knew her Charles enjoyed music; he often listened to a collection of holiday tunes recorded by Gloria, and once burst into song at a family Hanukkah celebration. But she was certain he had nothing that resembled talent. Charles was more like an autistic child than the social butterfly so often seen among Williams kids. He had trouble communicating, trouble looking people in the eye. In fourth grade, he became obsessed with *Toy Story* and made headway with his classmates by talking about Buzz Lightyear and Woody and all the toys that came to life in Andy's room in the movie; but when Charles was still gushing about Hamm and Bo Peep and Mr. Potato Head a year later, he didn't understand why he was being shut out by the other children. Kay had to explain that the boys were growing up, that they had enough of *Toy Story*, and, that they wanted to move on to something else. Sports was something that the kids could relate to, and something that Charles enjoyed. He plunged into reading and research, and soon Charles was a walking encyclopedia on Fenway Park and the Red Sox, had memorized the names of all the quarterbacks in the National Football League, and was constantly popping *History of Sports* videos into the

VCR. Kay sent Charles to music camp to make friends and to work on social skills, and nothing more.

Charles, now twelve, arrived at Belvoir Terrace in 1996, with Kay and a full-time aide in tow. Family-style meals were an important part of the camp experience, but Charles wanted no part of them. He was very picky and would only eat foods brought from home, packed in familiar plastic containers. Kay smuggled contraband food in for him. While more than one hundred people packed Belvoir's dining hall, passing dishes up and down the table, Charles nibbled from his own stash.

Camp director Nancy Goldberg watched Charles with a frown. She was a longtime observer of the delicate interplay between children and parents and felt she could spot trouble from a mile away. Kay had told Nancy that Charles was mainstreamed at school, but Nancy soon concluded that Charles wasn't so much "mainstreamed" as "babysat." Nancy marched up to Charles and told him to eat! Eat! Eat what everyone else was eating! Charles froze, and wouldn't eat anything at all.

Charles had a very hard time that first year at camp. All the new people, sounds, and sights seemed to overwhelm him, short-circuit him. He didn't participate, didn't sing when the others were singing, didn't dance when the others were dancing. Kay could tell he felt besieged, like a stunned deer in the headlights, but when she tried to talk to him about it he insisted he loved camp and was having a marvelous time.

Nancy pulled Kay aside. Kay clearly loved Charles, but her love was going to ruin him, Nancy warned. These people following him around, tending to his every need, were killing any gumption that he might have to do something for himself. Do you want Charles to spend the rest of his life as an infant, dependent on other people for everything? Or do you want him to be able to be all that he can be? Nancy suggested that it might be best if Charles left camp and tried again next year, when he was more ready.

Kay was shocked. She fought back tears. If she was younger, she might just have packed up and gone home and that would have been the end of that. But Kay refused to leave.

Charles tells me every hour how much he loves it here, she told Nancy. He's just overloaded. Give him a chance. Give us a chance.

Nancy acquiesced, and every day, Charles participated a little more. By the end of the week he was tested against the piano and was able to sing the notes back. Your son has perfect pitch, she was told.

Nancy told Kay to get Charles into singing lessons. He sang a little—not terribly well—but with some training, who knows, anything could happen. Nancy would help Kay find a voice teacher in her area who was willing to work with a special-needs child. But most important, Nancy said, let Charles grow up.

Charles didn't start his voice lessons learning kiddie songs. He went straight to show tunes and Broadway numbers. Slowly, surely, a decent baritone emerged. Kay would never forget the first time they harmonized together.

You have to understand that special-needs children take and take and take, Kay said. At some point, regular children learn to reciprocate, but special needs children can't. Charles started singing "Candle on the Water," a sentimental ballad from the Disney film *Pete's Dragon*: "I'll be your candle on the water, / My love for you will always burn . . ."

Kay started singing along, and their voices snapped together like lock and key in an achingly lovely harmony. At that moment, they connected in a way Kay had never known, and never expected. They looked each other right in the eye, and it sent chills up Kay's spine; for the first time, Charles had given her a gift, and he knew it. It was a transcendent moment, almost like a prayer. Music connected them, worked some magic, opened up a whole new world. Charles would probably never be as accomplished as

Gloria, but that was completely beside the point. It was the first time he found something that truly belonged to him, that he could do in a completely, delightfully, average way.

Camp was in session. Kay was sitting on a rock in front of the mansion. Gentle hills unfurled before her, a brilliant palette of green bristling with pines so stout and tall and straight they seemed like a royal army. Howard joined her, admiring the peaceful view.

Gloria really looks forward to this week all year long, he told her.

Charles is the same way, Kay said. The trees swayed in the breeze as the two started sharing their hearts. Their kids had such distinct, and bizarre, peaks and valleys. Stunning gifts and agonizing deficits that make them like precocious, eternal twelve-year-olds, in the world but not of it. They spoke about how easily people give up on kids like theirs, about how so little is asked of them. Howard's constant worry was what would happen to Gloria after he and Sylvia were gone. Who would make sure she continues her music lessons? That she stretches and grows artistically, trying new pieces and new styles? That she takes care of her health, gets to sing for people, is happy? It would be wonderful if something like the community born of this camp could be available for Williams people fifty-two weeks a year instead of only one, Howard said.

Kay had heard for years about Howard's dream of a music academy for Williams people, but she listened politely as he tailored the argument to her circumstances. Wouldn't it be marvelous if there was a place our kids could go after high school to really learn a skill, to do something they love, to become productive members of society? Kay would see, soon enough, the long, blank years that stretched after high school graduation, years they would try to fill with as much meaning as possible. But it was so hard. These Williams people were warehoused in menial jobs when they had such great musical potential. We owe it to them to tap that potential, Howard said. He had been on the verge of getting commitments from the University of California and the University of Texas to start residential music academies where Williams people could live together, make music together, and grow older together, but nothing ever seemed to go through. The Bernons had championed so many good causes over the years. Kay was such a pro at raising funds for worthy programs. And she had been on the board of the Williams Syndrome Foundation for years. Would she consider stepping up her commitment, and championing the cause of a music academy for Williams kids?

Kay stared off into the distant army of pines. What, indeed, did the future hold for Charles?

Before Bellugi left camp, she stuck her head into a gathering of parents. I'm convinced, she told Howard. *Finally*, Howard thought. Finally.

Once Levitin and Bellugi had returned to their labs, they set about analyzing the data they had gathered at Belvoir. The picnic table sessions, as they came to be known, weren't the most rigorously designed studies they had ever done, but some very interesting things happened there nonetheless.

In the end, they used responses from two girls and six boys from camp, ranging in age from nine to twenty. Now they needed a comparison group of regular kids so they could contrast results. They wanted educationally sophisticated kids who had at least three years of musical instruction. So they recruited eight from the highly rated public schools in Palo Alto—two females and six males, just like the Williams kids. All were taking private music lessons. They were matched for mental age, so they were a good deal younger than the Williams kids, ranging from five to seven. Levitin went to their homes, took the kids into their backyards, and had them repeat the same "echo clapping" exercises that the Williams kids had done at Belvoir's redwood picnic tables.

Now there were hours of tape to analyze and "grade." Levitin signed up two jazz musicians as "independent coders"—a drummer and a vocalist, who also played trumpet. They were "blind": They didn't know the hypotheses that Levitin and Bellugi were working with, and they didn't know which group had produced which samples. They'd just listen.

The coders were given simple instructions: mark each response as correct or incorrect. "Incorrect" was when a child clearly played a different rhythm than the presenter. The coders could make notes about the quality of the responses if they wanted. It took weeks.

The hypothesis Levitin and Bellugi had taken to Belvoir was that savants had proven to be good with melody and harmony but bad with rhythm, and they expected Williams people to have trouble keeping a beat as well. A similar test of developmentally disabled children had been done twenty years earlier and found them to be far worse at echo tapping than regular kids.

But that's not what Levitin and Bellugi found at all. To their surprise, the Williams people actually got slightly more right than the regular kids, though the difference wasn't statistically significant. Each group made errors about 31 percent of the time. It was astounding that, given their problems with eye-hand and spatial coordination, the Williams kids were able to control their bodies well enough to perform like this.

But what really caught Levitin's attention were the "qualifying notes" that the coders made as they listened to the tapes. When some of the kids were wrong, the coders said, they were often wrong in "interesting ways." Levitin asked them what that meant, and they said that, many times, when the kids didn't reproduce the rhythm perfectly, they clapped a rhythm that had a clear musical relationship to the original.

What, exactly, do you mean? Levitin asked.

One of the coders explained that "it sounds like a call-and-response; as though the subject is creating a musically logical completion to the rhythm provided."

Put more simply, some of the kids seemed to be making *music* out of their responses, rather than "slavishly mimicking the experimenter." It had the improvisational flow and feel of a jam session, the coders said.

Levitin and Bellugi asked both coders to go back, independently, and listen again to the responses they had marked as incorrect. Divide the incorrect responses into those that they felt were "elaborations or creative completions," and those that were clearly wrong. Again, they'd make their decisions "blind," without knowing which group they were grading.

The results were fascinating. The Williams kids were *three times* as likely to offer "creative completions"—that is, rhythmically compatible responses—as the regular kids were. And when wrong, the Williams kids seemed to have an innate understanding of what Levitin called "the rules of musical grammar;" their responses sounded finished. They had rhythmic resolution (the "two bits" part of "shave and a haircut, two bits") and fit the musical context far more often than the regular kids' wrong responses. The Williams kids also had flair; their embellishments fit the rhythm pattern and they carried complicated bits of syncopation over into their responses, "preserving the rhythm's global structure."

Williams kids did this 45 percent of the time, while regular kids did it only 15 percent of the time. And *everyone* in the Williams group was able to do it; there were no significant differences between them on their propensity to do creative completions. If the Williams kids were unable to replicate a rhythm, for whatever reason, they tended to err on the side of "rhythmic musicality," taking the larger musical context into account.

Their paper was published the following year in the journal *Music Perception*:

> For much of its history, experimental psychology has viewed intelligence as somewhat monolithic, and mental retardation as

reflecting more or less uniform impairment across the various domains of cognitive functioning. We report evidence for relatively preserved musical rhythm processing in individuals with Williams syndrome, supporting the theory that musical ability constitutes an independent intelligence.

Howard convinced Bellugi and researchers Paul Wang and Frank Greenberg to coauthor an article with him for *Scientific American*. Usually, pieces got into that magazine only after authors were invited to submit; Howard, however, didn't wait for any invitations. He pitched the story of Williams syndrome to an editor he met while working on the hydra, stressed the mysterious musicality of many Williams people, and was gratified when the piece was published in a six-page spread, featuring moody portraits of Brian draped pensively over his guitar, and of Gloria rapturously singing.

{chapter 13}
A PLACE FOR US

I n some parts of the world, music is not entertainment, but prayer. A way of talking to the gods and hearing the gods talk back. By surrendering to the power of music, it is said, one can experience the bliss of merging into the eternal "universal soul."

Intuitively, Williams people seem to grasp this transcendent relationship with sound. "When I play music, I feel love," said Mary Hendryx of Dallas, who composes her own songs on piano. "I feel warm. I don't feel scared at all. When I don't play music, I feel bored. I feel dead."

"Music is everlasting life," said Chris Lawson, the elegant pianist with the penchant for Scottish bagpipes. "It's soothing to your soul. When I play, I feel very energized, very excited."

The haunting beauty of a Gregorian chant sends tears streaming down Alec Sweazy's face. Music moves Tori Ackley to weep as well. "It's so beautiful, it really inspires me to be better at what I need to be better at," Tori said.

"It makes me blossom like a flower," said Kelley Martin.

This reverence is deeply felt, and Williams people were teaching it to those who loved them. It was the treasure Kay Bernon received from her son Charles. Music had been such a gift to both of them; Kay felt it let her glimpse inside his soul. Howard was right, Kay decided. Charles, and the others like him, deserved more opportunities to pursue their passion.

So it was with a deep sigh and a steely resolve that Kay Bernon decided to get down to business with the Williams Syndrome Foundation board. She had been hearing high-flying talk about a music academy for Williams people for as long as she could remember; now, the talk would turn into action. Kay had access to strata of society that the rest of the Williams families could only dream about, and she intended to employ every advantage she enjoyed to transform dream into reality.

In the snowy cold of January 1999, Kay organized a weekend retreat at a charming inn across the street from Belvoir Terrace in Lenox. Sharon was there. Nancy Goldberg and theater teacher Bryce Hill were there. So were Suzanne Hanser, chair of the Berklee College of Music's music therapy program; Nancy and Bruce Walsh of Canada, parents of singer Lisa Walsh; and Liz and Bob Costello, parents of singer Meghan Finn. And, in an effort to bridge the acrimonious divide between the Williams Syndrome Foundation and Association, association director Terry Monkaba was there. And of course Howard was there, even though it was his seventieth birthday. There was a cake, a copy of *Tuesdays With Morrie* (the book Mitch Albom wrote about the last days of his friend's life, which made Howard think, "Am I going to die?"), and a young lady who paused as Howard tried to open a door for her and proceeded, saying, "Age before beauty."

Bob Costello had succeeded Howard as president of the Williams Syndrome Foundation, and Bob and Liz presided at this meeting, urging everyone to dream. It was an intense meeting where competing visions battled for prominence: Would an academy concentrate on teaching Williams people the life skills they'd need to live on their own, as Bob and Liz so wanted? Or would it focus almost purely on music, as Howard wanted?

Should it be a permanent, year-round, residential community, as Howard so longed for? Or should it be more like a college, operating on a nine-month time frame and graduating its students in two or three years? Should it be a village, with housing for parents who wanted to stay close to their kids, as Howard wanted? Or should they start smaller, and think strictly in terms of independence for the students?

There was discussion and disagreement and creative tension. Howard sometimes had to leave the room to cool down. Kay coaxed everyone to find the middle ground, and after staying up into the wee hours, agonizing over words and clashing over visions, they concluded the school couldn't, shouldn't, be just a music academy. It had to help Williams kids tackle everyday, practical skills like cooking, going shopping, taking buses, balancing a checkbook. Things they would need to know if they were to have truly full and independent lives. And it would not be a year-round village; it would be on a traditional college schedule, with summers off.

They created a mission statement: *To build a residential, postsecondary school to provide comprehensive training in music, essential academics, social, vocational, and independent living skills. The school will offer a two-year certificate program to adults with cognitive disabilities who want to enhance their musical abilities. Music will have a central place in the school as an ability to be developed and a way to facilitate other kinds of learning. Graduates will earn "Certificates of Completion," with a concentration in either general studies or music and human service.*

They drew up a student profile: *The program is for the cognitively disabled adult, eighteen or older, who has demonstrated an ability in, or passion for, music, and wants to pursue his musical potential. The student should be motivated, emotionally stable, and in general good health. The program will include, but not be limited to, students with Williams syndrome.* (The fairest thing was to open the school up to all disabled musicians, they decided.)

They agreed on a philosophy: *The school will maximize each stu-*

dent's potential, building on strengths and remediating weaknesses in a nurturing and supportive environment. Music has a central place, as an ability to be developed and a way to facilitate other kinds of learning. Students will participate meaningfully in community life through volunteering and the formation of a musical troupe that will give public performances, as well as entertain at nursing homes, retirement homes, and elderly day-care sites.

And they agreed on a name: the Berkshire Hills Music Academy.

At the end of the weekend, Bryce Hill signed on as interim director, and immediately started scouting schools for the disabled so he could borrow the best ideas. Music and Minds, a pilot program at the University of Connecticut (begun at the instigation of Sally Reis, a cousin of pianist/bagpiper Chris Lawson's mother), was a logical place to start. Reis was an educational psychologist who specialized in teaching gifted children, and she thought the musical gifts of people like Chris could be used to strengthen their weak areas. Music and Minds used Williams people's deep love of music to teach everything from math to language. There were daily classes in chorus, music, movement, drama, and math. There were evening drum sessions, in-house musical nightclubs, field trips to hear and play the local carillon. Students lived in double rooms and ate in the university cafeteria.

"All participants displayed what may be described as a romance with music and rhythm," wrote the researchers, who included Audrey Don, the Canadian artist-turned-neuropsychologist who did the first study of music and Williams syndrome people. "The absence of music in their school experiences and sometimes in their home life resulted in the loss of opportunities to find and develop their potential talent areas and also to find joy in their lives. Music could be used as a powerful teaching tool throughout school years to help develop skills in deficit areas."

The researchers blasted mainstream educators for focusing on disabilities rather than trying to develop talents and use them to teach. "We must avoid the usual assessment stance of looking for disturbances or negative symptoms. While school psychologists are not usually inclined to look for positive behaviors, it is the positive behaviors that might act as a base to build constructive educational plans for this group," they wrote.

This would be a template upon which to build the new school. Bryce Hill started writing the curriculum and bearing down on the most practical and problematic question: Where?

Belvoir Terrace, Howard and the foundation board felt, was a logical site. Belvoir was closed from September to June, exactly when the academy would be in session, and was only used as a camp in the summer. Many potential students were familiar and comfortable with it. Kay and Bryce were excited at the possibility, and started negotiating.

If the academy renovated Belvoir into a year-round facility, it could stay rent-free for five years, Nancy said. There was no money yet, but Kay penciled things out: renovating Belvoir would cost some $500,000 to $1 million. Much less than it would cost to buy a building, but still a sizable chunk of change. And what would happen after those five years were up? It might be worth the investment if Nancy could promise that the school would be at Belvoir for the long term; but Nancy didn't feel she could make a promise like that. Who knew if the camp would still be in the family in ten, fifteen, twenty years? And Nancy also had liability to worry about. The legal documents that were drawn up caused discomfort all around, and the founders decided they'd best look elsewhere.

A lovely property down the road from Belvoir Terrace soon came up for sale. Kay and Bryce plunged into more negotiations, but the site was bound up in a financial scandal involving a non-profit music foundation, so that didn't pan out either. Disappointed and frustrated, they decided that they were probably limiting themselves by restricting their search to Lenox. True, the town was lovely, Belvoir was there, and Tanglewood was nearby, but that was all summer activity. Nothing much happened in Lenox during the fall, winter, and spring, when the academy would be in session. There really wasn't any reason the academy had to be in Lenox at all.

Howard had always hoped the academy would be affiliated with a college or university. It would give the Williams students access to real campus life and regular role models, as well as good teachers and willing interns. In return, the university's researchers would get access to some of the most interesting scientific subjects in the world. And there was certainly no shortage of colleges in the Northeast, where Kay had her most solid base of support. So they broadened their horizons: Kay would target every educational institution within a hundred-mile radius of Lenox.

She wrote dozens of letters detailing the grand mission of the academy, the great mysteries of Williams syndrome, and how beneficial a collaboration could be to all. She mailed the letters off and waited. And waited. She received only one response: from the University of Massachusetts, where she had a friend on the board of trustees. Her friend called the vice chancellor and talked up the proposal; now the university was interested and wanted to meet to flesh things out.

It's a good thing, Kay would later say, that she didn't know what she was doing. She soon found herself at a long conference table with smart-suited administrators and distinguished scientists from the Five Colleges—Amherst, Hampshire, Mount Holyoke, and Smith Colleges, and the University of Massachusetts, Amherst. They wanted to know more about the academy and the syndrome and how a partnership would work. With Howard "attending" by teleconference, Kay showed video, cited studies, and painted a picture of what they envisioned. Howard, his voice tinny but intense through the telephone speaker, talked up all the research possibilities and got the scientists excited. Howard had urged Kay to get the curriculum vitae for everyone in attendance so they'd have an idea who they were dealing with, and Kay left the meeting weighed down with hundreds of pages. Later, as she eagerly thumbed through them, her eyes widened. These were people who had received millions in grant money from the National Institutes of Health. They would be invaluable collaborators.

Soon, Kay invited the Lenhoffs to meet the provost and scientists of the University of Massachusetts. Howard knew the school pretty well—he once was a candidate for dean of its graduate school, and a former student was on the faculty. Provost Cora Marrett said she saw how an academy could help researchers; once Gloria sang Otis Redding's "Dock of the Bay," Marrett broke into a big smile, and it was clear she saw how it could help the Williams people, too.

Sharon Libera once taught at one of the Five Colleges—Mount Holyoke in South Hadley—and soon learned that Mount Holyoke might sell "the Orchards," the grand Skinner estate bequeathed to it in 1946. Joseph Skinner built the sprawling mansion on forty acres in 1915 and made it one of the finest homes of its time, with twenty-three rooms, soaring ceilings, finely carved staircases, and soothing mountain views through walls of west-facing windows. The Skinner fortune was made in fine silk mills, and Joseph's thinking was far ahead of his time: his strong belief in education for women led him to became president of Mount Holyoke's board of trustees, and when he died, he left the Orchards to the college. His daughter lived there for decades. It was home to a corporate executive and the National Yiddish Book Center. And now, nearly eighty-five years after it was built, it was in great need of care. Restoration, though, would be too expensive an endeavor for the college.

Sharon lived just a few miles away, and drove out to investigate. She took one glimpse at the mansion, framed by trees like Tara in *Gone with the Wind*, and knew it was the place. Paint was dull, windows were dirty, and the whole place smelled musty, but she could see the tired bedrooms transformed into dormitories. She could see parlors turned into classrooms and practice rooms. She could see the grand living room, which had hosted music recitals so long ago, brought back to life as a welcoming place where students could gather at night. Kay instantly fell in love as well. We will buy this house, they both vowed. They just had to raise $2 million to pay for it.

The mission became all consuming for Kay. She spent ten hours a day making phone calls, writing letters, and asking friends to donate time and money. Her passion was visceral, and everyone heard it in her voice; even if they didn't have disabled children, they understood that all parents wanted their children to have a place where they could fit in, where they could be their very best. The Berkshire Hills Music Academy soon filed incorporation papers as a nonprofit, and Kay became president of its board. Her brother-in-law, Boston philanthropist Alan Bernon, would be treasurer. They declared that their ideal property was the Skinner estate in South Hadley, Massachusetts.

Armed with a blueprint, Kay started working. She organized a party in her elegant home on Nantucket Island, invited many wealthy friends and neighbors, and asked the Lenhoffs to attend so Gloria could sing. Kay hired a professional accompanist, ordered sophisticated sound equipment that had to be delivered from Boston, and drove down to the ferry with Howard to pick it up. Together, they wrestled it into the truck. Guests started arriving and Howard marveled at their attire: Women wore designer dresses and Nantucket "basket jewelry" of gold and silver that harkened back to the weavings done by sailors and fishermen a century ago to pass the time. Most of the men wore blue sport jackets and brown khaki trousers, which Howard reluctantly mimicked. One rebellious man in a flowing white shirt caught Howard's eye; he looked interesting, so Howard introduced himself and learned that the man was a musician with Aerosmith. Howard had never heard of Aerosmith. Oh yes, Howard said, I read that book by Sinclair Lewis. The book was *Arrowsmith*; it had nothing to do with Aerosmith; and Howard had no idea he had just met rocker Brad Whitford. The conversation ended on a funny note, and Howard moved on.

Kay's husband was smoking a cigar. Howard had to object: The smoke would make Gloria cough and impact her singing voice. It also made Howard nauseous. Kay quickly asked her husband to extinguish the cigar, and then asked for everyone's attention. She introduced Howard, who gave a brief overview of Gloria's life and of Williams syndrome, and then Gloria launched into "Mi Chiamano Mimi" from Puccini's *La Bohème*. In Italian she sang: "I live by myself, all alone, / in my little white room / I look upon the roofs and the sky / But when the thaw comes / the first warmth of the sun is mine / the first kiss of April is mine!" Sylvia nudged Howard and motioned to the man in the flowing white shirt: he was weeping. After Gloria finished her five songs, Brad Whitford and wife, Karen, hurried to Howard and Sylvia and told them how deeply moved they were. Whitford would love it if Gloria would learn his song, "I Don't Want to Miss a Thing" from the movie *Armageddon*, and sing it. "I could spend my life in this sweet surrender / I could stay lost in this moment forever / Every moment spent with you / Is a moment I treasure. . . ." Gloria smiled and said she'd be happy to learn it.

With that success under her belt, Kay started work on the first fund-raiser. She had ducked into a coffee shop in Lenox for some fuel when she ran into a music teacher from Belvoir Terrace — Franco Spoto, a tenor who was one of Gloria's favorite voice teachers at camp. Kay told Spoto about the plans for Berkshire Hills, lamented about how much money she had to raise, and wistfully said that it would be nice if one of the well-known local musicians donated a performance for the fund-raiser. It just so happened that Spoto's wife gave horseback-riding lessons to violinist Lucia Lin, wife of Boston Pops conductor Keith Lockhart. Lockhart had met the Williams campers one summer when they had attended a Boston Pops rehearsal. Spoto would pass the word on. The worst Lockhart and Lin could say was no.

Soon Kay got a phone call from Keith Lockhart's secretary. Who? the disbelieving Kay asked three times. Lockhart had heard about her efforts, was 100 percent behind her, and had a string of dates to suggest for the fund-raiser. Really? Kay kept saying. Are you sure?

Kay hit the phones again with ferocity. She had to convince a hotel in Boston to donate a ballroom. She had to convince Tiffany & Co. to underwrite invitations and provide gifts for the guests. She had to draw up a guest list including every captain of industry and fountain of philanthropy and creative artist she knew. With a gulp, she set the ticket price at $1,000 a head. "The Founders Dinner," she would call it, 1999.

Kay was uncommonly nervous as the Ritz Carlton ballroom began to fill. Keith Lockhart and wife Lucia Lin gave a forty-five-minute performance, and after dinner Gloria sang Bocelli's "Con Te Partiro" with Franco Spoto and Delibes' "The Flower Duet" from *Lakme* with Jacqueline Zander of the Boston Lyric Opera. Stephen Lord, opera director, accompanied them. Lockhart had said he could only stay until 8 PM, but he was there to close the doors when things broke up at nearly midnight. Boston rocker Brad Whitford of Aerosmith was there as well. Gloria astounded him, he said. Her courage and her passion for music moved him deeply.

"It became overwhelmingly clear to me that music is a common language, no matter who you are," he later said, and agreed to help raise awareness, and money, for this daring new academy. He introduced the Williams musicians to his Aerosmith cohort, Tom Hamilton, and Hamilton signed onto the effort as well. They agreed to be the headliners at the next benefit for the Berkshire Hills Music Academy.

The Founders Dinner raised $1 million. Kay's family kicked in another $1 million. Now, they had enough to buy the Skinner estate.

Kay was flush with triumph and panic as she signed the purchase agreement with Mount Holyoke College. The dream that they had dreamed seemed like it was actually going to come true, and there were few things more thrilling and terrifying than that. But owning the mansion was only half the battle; now she had to raise enough money to renovate and restore the main house, as well as build an addition with music rooms and classrooms and computer labs and dormitories and a public performance space. Kay took a deep breath, pulled out her Rolodex, and got back to work.

When Bryce Hill decided to step down as interim director for personal reasons, the small circle of founders agonized over who would replace him. They thought of the staff at the University of Connecticut's Music and Minds program — a template for how Berkshire Hills would teach — and called Greg Williams, who was its music director. Williams was working on his PhD in music education from the University of Connecticut and was forever changed by working with Williams people. "That ten-day experience absolutely changed how I taught," Williams said. "It made me ask, 'How do I really connect with this person? What is this person good at?' I rediscovered some of the joy I'd found making music when I was young." He agreed to sign on and make Berkshire Hills a reality.

The "honorary committee" is a useful tool when fund-raising. The luminaries who agree to be on it invariably become committed patrons and generous donors. Kay employed all her contacts, Nancy Goldberg's contacts, Howard's contacts, and their contacts' contacts, until they put together an honorary committee that would read like an extremely eclectic Who's Who of music: Victor Borge; Placido Domingo; Itzhak Perlman and wife, Toby; Aerosmith members Tom Hamilton and wife, Terry; Brad Whitford and wife, Karen. Kay set the date for the next fund-raiser, orchestrated an infinite string of details ("9 a.m., stage constructed . . . piano arrives by 11 a.m. from Steinert Piano Co. Piano will be tuned by noon and placed on the left side of the 12 by 24 stage. Angle the piano so the audience can see Mr. Borge's hands. Keep in mind the stage will also include the Aerosmith setup — guitar, bass drums . . ."), and on November 18, 2000, in an elegant ballroom at the Ritz-Carlton Hotel in Boston,

Williams musicians took the stage with Aerosmith's two head-liners. Brad Whitford played guitar, Tom Hamilton played bass, Canadian drummer Jason Dennis played drums, and Gloria played accordion on Whitford's "I Don't Want to Miss a Thing"— the song Whitford asked Gloria to sing the very first time he met her. Before they slid into "Sweet Emotion," Hamilton joked with the well-dressed crowd: "Moshing is encouraged, but for those who prefer not to mosh, just rattle your jewelry." They stormed into the hard-rocking song and Jason Dennis reached such a fever pitch during his drum solo that a drumstick flew from his hand. He kept the beat steady with the other hand as Whitford hastily retrieved his stick; when it was over, Whitford again had tears in his eyes, and the entire crowd gave Jason a standing ovation. Jason called it one of the highlights of his life.

Ben Monkaba, son of Williams Syndrome Association director Terry Monkaba, took over the drum set for an explosive version of "Come Together" as Terry proudly looked on. He was good. Williams people really *do* have an uncanny ability to learn, and excel, at music, she thought.

The concert ended with Franco Spoto and Gloria singing the "Drinking Song" duet from Verdi's *La Traviata*—a corny segue to the cocktail hour. A New Orleans–style parade led by John Libera on clarinet and Greg Williams on trumpet paraded everyone out of the ballroom to a rousing version of "When the Saints Go Marching In." Guests sipped cocktails to music by Tori, Meghan, John, Ben, and others. There was a silent auction, and then dinner. Victor Borge played after the meal—one of his last US concerts—and everything wrapped up with students carrying candle-top flashlights and singing "Somewhere" from *West Side Story*. Somewhere, they sang. Somehow. Someday.

Guests pulled many tissues from their pockets and purses that night. In the end, the event raised another $1 million, enough to help transform the Skinner mansion into the Berkshire Hills Music Academy. Perhaps somewhere, somehow, someday had arrived.

{chapter 14}

PROOF

Maggie Hosseini sat on the porch of her Maryland home with her grandmother, watching as the other neighborhood teens got ready for the high school prom. They exchanged corsages and boutonnieres, primped for pictures, then drove off in shiny cars to the storied party they'd remember for the rest of their lives. Maggie was not going. Kids in her special education program didn't usually attend the prom, and no one had invited her anyway.

Grammie, Maggie said, I wonder, sometimes, how it would be if I were normal.

Her grandparents' hearts ached for her. Williams people understand they are different, grandfather Bill Crow said. They understand their limitations. It breaks your heart.

They tried to cheer up Maggie by pointing out that soon she'd be heading off to Massachusetts on an adventure far greater than any prom: Maggie would be a member of the inaugural class at the Berkshire Hills Music Academy, the first residential academy in America dedicated to the musicianship of cognitively impaired people. She would live away from home for the first time, with people just like herself for the first time, learning to be independent, studying something she enjoyed, charting a course for her future.

Maggie had always liked music, but she didn't show much proclivity for it; her grandparents had met Howard and Gloria at conferences, saw the *60 Minutes* piece shortly before Maggie's eighteenth birthday, and decided to make a week at Belvoir's music camp a gift to Maggie, just so she'd have something special to do. That was only three summers ago. Maggie sang for the first time at camp, started taking singing lessons at home, and her self-confidence blossomed. Now, who knows what the future might hold? She wasn't Maria Callas, but she loved singing and was willing to work hard to make herself better. The music academy was a wish granted.

Though Berkshire Hills was set to open in just one month, it was still a construction site. An army of painters, carpenters, electricians, plumbers, and drywall installers swarmed over the grounds, madly trying to prepare for its first class of fourteen in September of 2001. The transformation of the main house was well under way, but the new addition, six thousand square feet of classrooms, music rooms, computer labs, and dormitories, still bristled with naked two-by-fours. Howard, Kay, and Sharon, taking a field trip from the eighth annual Williams music camp at Belvoir Terrace, toured the construction nervously. It seemed impossible that it would be ready on time.

Sharon's son John was going to be in the inaugural class as well, and he used this time at camp to try new things. In a familiar practice room at Belvoir Terrace he snapped together his clarinet, tugged on the brim of his baseball cap, and pushed his aviator glasses higher on his nose. His teacher arranged the score to a Mozart minuet on the black iron music stand and he took his seat before it. Sheet music was sheer formality for most Williams musicians, but not for John. He could now sight-read.

"This is a minuet," teacher Heather Johnson said as John surveyed the score. "A minuet. What kind of piece is that?"

John stared at the music, silently rocking in time to a beat only he could hear.

"Like the 'Macarena'?" Johnson offered, trying to coax him

down a logical pathway. "What do you do with the 'Macarena'?" She waited. "The 'Macarena'?" She bounced in her chair, doing all the 'Macarena' moves. "You dance to it!" she finally cried. "This is like an old 'Macarena'!"

John smiled with understanding, then lifted the clarinet to his lips and began to play. Squinting slightly, he translated the marks on the page into music—something that, in the world of Williams, was like flying. Mozart's minuet is coy and playful, sprightly and quick, but John played it even faster than that, notes tumbling out like words in a breathless story that couldn't be told quickly enough. He ended in a flurry of flashy trills, fingers fluttering on silver keys as he made the last notes warble like lovestruck birds.

"Good, good!" Johnson said as John resumed his body bop. "Your rhythm is perfect and I can hear the clarity of each note. But they didn't do it as quickly as you did it right now. Just think how the ladies would be tripping over those big skirts!" John smiled again.

"Once more," Johnson said, "and ease up on those trills."

This time, she set the pace. John fell into step instantly. He played with ease, unhurried, as the minuet unfolded. His tone was jaunty and clear, confident and cool, and the trills took on a more unaffected air.

"Great job!" Johnson said as the last warble faded away. "He reads very well," she said as an aside. "The other kids have to do it all by ear, but he has both things going. He really understands rhythmic structure."

When the lesson was over, John exited out the wrong door and froze in the foyer. He had been in that room dozens of times over the past eight years of camp, and was usually far better with directions than most Williams people, but still he was confused about where he was and where he was going. Johnson rushed out and gently redirected him to his next class. Thankful, and a bit rattled, John shuffled off to his saxophone lesson, just up the hill.

Johnson shook her head. This same young man was about to

start advanced studies at the Berkshire Hills Music Academy. "It's a rare, weird thing that has neurologically happened to these kids," she said. "And that's a wonderful thing to work with."

Johnson would know. Her daughter, Nora, had Williams syndrome as well.

A few miles away, scientists were gathering at the University of Massachusetts, Amherst, to mark the opening of Berkshire Hills and expose the Five Colleges faculty to the fundamentals of Williams syndrome. Daniel Levitin and Ursula Bellugi were there. Melissa (Thomas) Rowe and Helen Tager-Flusberg were there. Howard was there, as were Sharon, Terry Monkaba, and other parents from camp. The scientists would discuss brain organization, cognition and personality, language development, empathy, and, of course, music.

Howard usually took the podium for his scientific presentations with the excitement of a schoolboy. This time, it was different. He was nervous. He, a biochemist by training, was about to deliver his findings on absolute pitch and Williams syndrome to a group of psychologists and music researchers. Well, he figured, drumming up his courage, the psychologists and music researchers would probably be just as uncomfortable speaking to a room full of biochemists. He took a deep breath and began.

Everyone knew Howard. He had been hounding many of them for more than a decade to investigate music and Williams. But he started from the beginning, as if he were a total stranger. His biochemistry background. How he didn't mean to get into cognitive research. How it just, sort of, happened. "I thought my daughter was unique because she was my daughter," he said, eliciting chuckles. "But as we met parents and teachers, I became convinced that many others had musical talents. And I have yet to meet the Williams person who has stage fright, no matter what degree of talent they have. Give them a microphone and their whole personality is transformed."

Howard had one goal when he started his research: to quantify absolute pitch in Williams people. He knew that a third of the Williams parents he met believed their kids had absolute pitch — that rare ability to hear a solitary note and know it's a G, or an A, or a B-flat, without hearing it in relation to any other musical tones. He explained how his research assistant, Ole Perales, traveled all over the country to test five Williams musicians. A correct answer earned one point. Answers off by a half tone earned three-quarters of a point. Answers off by a full tone or more earned zero points.

To provide the contrast, two groups of controls were selected. All were university graduates. Most everyone in the first group had some musical training; those in the second group were serious musicians working on master's of fine arts degrees in music.

The results, he said, were staggering. Absolute pitch appeared to be at least *ten times* more prevalent in the Williams population than in the regular population.

Previous studies found that about one in every *ten thousand* has absolute pitch. Howard and his colleagues concluded that, at a minimum, about one in every *one thousand* Williams people has absolute pitch. Eyebrows raised. He explained how he arrived at that number: there are about five thousand diagnosed Williams people in the United States and Canada. He tested five of them, and all had absolute pitch. That's one out of one thousand. In reality, the number was probably much higher: His analysis assumed that only the five he tested had absolute pitch. Clearly, there were others.

Of the five Williams people tested, all had near "ceiling-level ability," which is to say, they were correct the overwhelming amount of the time. There were 1,084 trials, and they were correct 97.5 percent of the time. The lowest scorer on one of the tests, he said, was Gloria — and she always scored at least 90 percent.

Howard had probed the literature on absolute pitch and developed a rationale explaining why it was so prevalent in Williams people. In the general population, it usually occurred only in people trained in music while very young—before age six. After that critical period, a window seemed to close in the brain of regularly developing folks. Anyone older than seven trying to develop absolute pitch would have a hard time, the experts said.

But, for some reason, that window didn't seem to close for Williams people, Howard said. Four of the five Ole tested didn't start their musical training until they were much older than six, and yet they still had absolute pitch. That led Howard and his colleagues to propose that the window of opportunity was jammed open somehow for Williams people, and probably remained open for life.

A number of researchers have concluded that we're all born with absolute pitch, and that it's important in acquiring language. That makes sense, since more than half of humankind speaks tonal languages, such as Mandarin, Vietnamese, or Thai, Howard said. It would also make sense that, once the language is learned and the ability is not needed anymore, it disappears.

Howard, Hickok, and Perales published two papers, one in a book titled *Toward a Theory of Neuroplasticity*, the other in the journal *Music Perception*. Their research showed that Williams people have a higher incidence of absolute pitch than do normal people, score higher in tests for absolute pitch than trained musicians who claim to have absolute pitch, and can acquire absolute pitch at an age when normal people can no longer do so.

"Our results demonstrate that, despite limitations in many areas of cognition, the five WS people in this study scored extremely well in over one thousand trials for AP, averaging as a group close to 98 percent correct," they wrote. "Their overall score compares favorably not only to that of our control participants, who scored 18 percent, but also to the performance of normal trained musicians who claimed to possess AP, who as a group scored 84.3 percent correct. . . . Thus, our results clearly demonstrate that an exceptional musical talent can be developed in spite of limitations in other cognitive domains, suggesting some degree of modularity in cognitive development in WS."

The comparison with trained musicians was especially impressive, Howard felt. It showed that the five Williams musicians tested better than all the trained musicians reported in the literature over a twenty-one-year period.

Levitin and Bellugi were up next, describing ongoing experiments supporting the view that Williams syndrome people are more engaged with musical activities than others, demonstrate earlier musical interest and ability than others, and tend toward greater musical creativity, both melodically and rhythmically, than others. Williams brains may be wired differently than the brains of regular people, they said, based on findings that Williams people use different neural circuitry than regular people when listening to music and noise.

Howard, Levitin, and Bellugi fielded questions from their colleagues. Some still disagreed with them. One wondered if Howard got such good results because he tested Williams people who he already knew had strong musical abilities.

Good question, Howard said. His five subjects were indeed the cream of the music camp's crop, but he had no alternative if he hoped to have quantitative results. Those five were the only ones who could name notes. He looked at it this way: The research did, indeed, show the maximum abilities in absolute pitch that Williams people were capable of achieving; but psychologists often designed studies that way. If you wanted to find out how fast a human being could run, you'd study Olympic athletes, not local community joggers, he reasoned.

There was also an undergraduate student who had done random tests of Williams children that were never published, who didn't think they had any more musical ability than regular children, though he had no doubt that the Williams kids were intensely attracted to music.

Howard said that trying to find outstanding ability in a

random group of Williams people was missing the point. He never said Williams people showed miraculous ability without any training; his point was that there was a mysteriously preserved pathway in the Williams brain that somehow made it possible for them to possess absolute pitch, to *learn* music and learn it well, and to retain complex pieces for uncanny lengths of time, even when they couldn't learn things that were far simpler. That, he felt, was what researchers missed by looking for ability in Williams children who didn't have any training and hadn't done any serious practicing. Howard knew one wouldn't find it there.

Some scientists capped the meeting with a trip to Belvoir Terrace to see the music camp's grand finale, and Alec Sweazy surely settled the argument for them. Alec, the baby who had matched tones as his mom played piano, loped to center stage, plopped onto the bench, and slid into position before an elegant grand piano. He ran his hands through his mop of blond hair, stretched his spindly arms toward the keyboard, and announced, "I'm going to play Prelude in C-sharp Minor by Rachmaninoff."

There was an audible intake of breath. The Prelude is a difficult piece, brimming with the brashness of a nineteen-year-old Rachmaninoff. Disjointed, episodic, varying wildly in tone and texture, it's a technically taxing work that Rachmaninoff came to despise. Rachmaninoff had had gigantic hands that made the Prelude easier to play; Alec, just sixteen, did not.

Alec lunged at the piano and pounded out dark, massive, menacing chords. There was silence; then torrents of furious notes that smashed into stillness and emerged, delicate and lyrical, on the other side. The music was soft as snow, then loud as thunder; slow as sunrise, then fast as flight. With a power that seemed far beyond his sixteen years, Alec executed a fierce tour de force, and his audience was suspended between awe and disbelief.

"That was the piece, the real piece, the whole piece, unabridged," whispered jazz pianist Mike Schiffer, who had been teaching Alec at camp for many summers. "And when you realize that he had to learn it all by ear, by rote, by watching his teacher, it truly blows your mind."

Alec can't read music, Schiffer said. He had tested him. But Alec has note-to-note, perfect recall of things he learned years ago. Schiffer knew he couldn't do that.

Alec grinned widely as the applause exploded. This was the same boy who was flummoxed by the intricacies of operating a can opener.

Berkshire Hills was going to open in just a few hours, making history as America's first residential college for mentally disabled musicians. But its windows were dirty. As carpenters and painters continued working on the addition, Kay, Bryce, and a few others raced through the main house with Windex and wads of paper towels, madly spraying and wiping, so the new students could see the glorious landscape.

Maggie Hosseini, John Libera, and their classmates rode into the academy's circular drive with bulging suitcases and butterflies in their stomachs on that warm September day. Trees draped around the mansion like protective arms. An angel fountain gurgled in the roundabout. And screeches of delight erupted as students greeted one another and their teachers with bear hugs and high fives, sharing the raw thrill of starting something entirely, unthinkably new. The mansion's addition still wasn't finished, but no one cared. The fourteen students were from nine states and two Canadian provinces, most of them Belvoir Terrace regulars who had harmonized together for years and were already great friends, like Tori Ackley, Brian Johnson, Chris Lawson, John, and Maggie. Only twelve of them had Williams; one had Down syndrome and the other an undiagnosed disability. But all of them loved music. The program was pricey: tuition and fees ran some twenty-five thousand dollars a year. Many students got help from public school districts, vocational training programs, foundation grants, or state mental retardation departments. Others paid out of pocket.

The students paired up with their new roommates, unpacked their bags, and, with ceremonial flourish, received their keys. They were simple metal keys, but they were loaded with symbolism: they marked the beginning of the road toward new, more independent lives. Tori Ackley pocketed her key, turned to her father, Bob, and said, "This is the happiest day of my life."

For Howard and Sylvia, it was a bittersweet victory. Berkshire Hills wasn't everything Howard had envisioned—he still wished for a year-round, residential community for Williams people—but here, Williams syndrome kids had a chance. Music could be their bridge to more independent futures, to fulfillment and acceptance in a wider world. Howard's armchair observations had translated into surprising science—science that may have changed the world for John, for Tori, for all the Williams students who would follow.

Gloria would not attend Berkshire Hills. She was forty-six. The academy was geared to college-aged people. It would only be in session nine months a year. Gloria needed a year-round home. Gloria needed more advanced musical training than the academy would offer, at least for a while. Berkshire Hills may have been largely her father's vision, but it was for the next generation. Not for her.

The academy was a grand experiment, and everybody knew it. Days began with group meetings at 8 AM, where they'd discuss everything from how to avoid colds and treat dry skin to homesickness and roommate conflicts. Then classes began, unlike classes they'd have found most anywhere else.

In computer class, students sorted through Internet offers from a "free CD" record club as the teacher pressed them to figure out the hidden costs. In practical math class, they opened bank accounts, got their own ATM cards, and practiced how to manage their own money. Social skills classes drilled them on the importance of personal boundaries, who it's OK to hug and not to hug, how to have a more healthy skepticism of strangers. There were English and public-speaking classes and one-on-one instruction on how to do laundry, cook, shop for groceries, get through the checkout line, and check for correct change. Everything was broken down into dozens of the most minute steps, from how to sort laundry to how much clothing to put in the machine to how to measure soap and turn the dials. There were also yoga classes and a fully equipped gym to work out any frustrations.

Afternoon classes were awash in music. Practice rooms pulsed and quivered with the fluid tone of a clarinet, the gentle tinkle of a piano, the liquid rush of vocal scales. There were classes in "how to be a music aide," covering the finer points of performing in daycare and senior citizens' centers, which they were required to do every week as part of their training. There were performance and musical theater classes as well.

Evenings were filled with free-form music. Before dinner, someone would park at the piano while the others crowded around to sing along; after dinner, a jazz ensemble gathered in the common room and jammed. John Libera especially loved the jazz jams; they challenged him, made him stretch, and made him start to feel like he was a real musician. Sharon was thrilled just to see him hanging around campus, talking with friends, having a genuine college experience. It was a simple pleasure she thought he would never know.

There were rough spots. Being away from home and family and all that was familiar was hard. Roommates quarreled over space and messes and chores. There were tears and fights and make-up sessions as the students shared emotional ups and downs and waded into the prickly waters of compromise and conflict resolution. But in addition to the usual complications attendant to living away from home for the first time, Berkshire Hills had something else, something that could be called the "prima donna problem." So many of the students had been musical stars in the Williams world; they hadn't been asked to blend in with a group for any serious length of time. They weren't used to critical reviews of their musical work, and when they learned they weren't perfect, some found it very hard to take.

"It's like I have twenty stars and have to make a constellation," program director Greg Williams told a journalist. "They need to learn when to retreat into the background, because in employment settings they won't always be stars, either."

Tori called her parents nearly every night to fill them in on her day, ask about how the dogs were doing, hear the latest news from home. But she wouldn't have traded Berkshire Hills for anything. In high school, she said, people teased her and told her she wasn't good at anything. At Berkshire Hills, people treated her with respect for who she was and made her feel good about herself.

"When I'm here, it seems like I'm in a family that has the same disabilities as me," she said. "We all have the same interests. We love each other no matter what. . . . They're the best friends I could ever ask for."

Tori's parents, Bob and Mandy Ackley, felt that the most important thing about Berkshire Hills was that it made Tori happy. If she ended up finding a job involving music, and living at least partially independently, that would be icing on the cake. They watched Tori blossom: her self-confidence soared, and she was more comfortable making decisions for herself.

Brian Johnson, the songwriter whose spontaneity so stunned researcher Dan Levitin, had finally found a home as well. "We all feel like we belong here," he said. "Without that, we wouldn't know where to turn."

Slowly the Berkshire Hills staff raised the bar higher. They asked the students to be more critical of themselves and taught them how to be more thoughtfully critical of others. Soon a two-track curriculum developed: one in performance, the other in music and human service. Boyfriend-girlfriend pairings blossomed, and staffers found themselves teaching the basics of human sexuality in addition to music and math.

"For a long time, our kids fell through the cracks because they learn so differently compared to the regular population, and even to the special-needs population," Williams Syndrome Association director Terry Monkaba said. "But now we're educating the educators, and Berkshire Hills is a great example of what's possible."

The academy's week ended on Friday afternoons with reflective rap sessions. Students sat in a circle and shared the highs and lows of the week. One Friday, Tori talked about a weekend spent at her parents' house, the dreariness of being treated like a little kid again, and the utter relief of returning to Berkshire Hills. "I came through that door on Monday and said, 'Boy, I'm glad to be home,'" she said. Her classmates erupted in cheers.

{chapter 15}

PROFESSIONAL PINNACLE

This was going to be different than the benefit concerts Gloria usually gave. She would not be pulling out her tried-and-true solo pieces. Instead, she would be the featured soloist with the sixty-five-piece San Diego Tifereth Israel Community Orchestra and the hundred-voice San Diego Master Chorale. Conductor David Amos, who had recorded off-the-beaten-track pieces with the London Symphony Orchestra, the Israel Philharmonic, the Royal Philharmonic, the Polish Radio Orchestra, and more, wanted Gloria to stretch. So he offhandedly suggested to Howard that Gloria consider doing Samuel Barber's oratorio, *Knoxville, Summer of 1915*, one of the most complex and challenging works in the modern repertoire.

The text was written by James Agee, a poet smitten with jazz improvisation, who strove for the jive of a jam session with words. The result was a prose poem taking a child's-eye view of a typical summer night in a typical backyard:

> . . . It has become that time of evening when people sit on their porches, rocking gently and talking gently and watching the street and the standing up into their sphere of possession of the trees, of birds' hung havens, hangars.

It was a gruelingly difficult work, conductor Amos admitted. Composer Barber said the text reminded him perfectly of his own childhood in Pennsylvania, and he set it to music that was sweetly nostalgic one second, and filled with yearning and pain the next; evoking calm and cool night air one second, and the "iron moan" of a passing streetcar the next. The pacing was jagged: As the words reflected the child's suddenly shifting train of thought, so did the music. Its unusual rhythms, awkward melodic intervals, and stream-of-consciousness text would push the memory of any soprano at any professional level, conductor Amos said. It was known as a lovely piece to listen to, and a dastardly difficult one to sing.

The benefit concert would be for a daycenter for adults with developmental disabilities in the dry hills of eastern San Diego County. It was named for a nineteenth-century French nun, St. Madeleine Sophie Barat, and was dedicated to helping the disabled reach their full potential in the wider community. It seemed only logical, then, that Gloria strive for something grander than anything she had attempted before.

Howard called Gloria's retired voice teacher, Barbara Hasty, and asked if she could help. Oh, Howard, Barbara said. That is such a phenomenally difficult piece. It's so rhythmically challenging. I'd have to work long and hard to sing that successfully myself.

But Howard was insistent. She can do it, he said. I really think she can do it.

Deep in her heart, Barbara was thinking, *never in a million years*. But if he was so set on having her try, the least she could do was help Gloria as much as she could. OK, I'll do everything I can, she said, but I don't know, Howard. I just don't know.

The piece is some twenty minutes long. Gloria worked for weeks on the smallest parts. Howard and Sylvia helped her enunciate and understand Agee's complicated lyrics. She listened to a recording of *Knoxville* again and again, and when it was finally time to rehearse with the full orchestra and chorale, conductor Amos wasn't sure what he had gotten them all into.

It did not go well. The version of *Knoxville* that Gloria had committed to memory used a very different pace and rhythm than Amos was using with the orchestra. With just two weeks to go before the performance, Gloria had to unlearn what she had learned, get a new recording of *Knoxville* that matched Amos's tempo—this one by soprano Dawn Upshaw—and commit it all to memory. The conductor of the San Diego Master Chorale spent hours with her in a one-on-one help session, and after that, Gloria felt she was ready.

At the next rehearsal, when Gloria opened her mouth and sang the first phrases, "We are talking now of summer evenings in Knoxville Tennessee in that time that I lived there so successfully disguised to myself as a child," Amos breathed a sigh of relief. Gloria had learned the new version inside and out. She was flexible, adjusting to the accompaniment of the full symphony orchestra and Amos's dancing baton. She could even be assertive to the point of stopping Amos and suggesting different tempos. Amos was impressed not only by the accuracy of her performance, but also by her musicality and enthusiasm. Gloria, he said, was an inspiration both to him and to the orchestra.

The day of the performance, Gloria settled into a dressing room in the performing arts center. It had a shower and a star on the door. She applied her makeup, ran through some warm-ups, and emerged on stage in a glittering gown, beaming with confidence. About twenty minutes later, when the piece was done, she bowed deeply and the audience rose to its feet. As applause thundered, she extended her arms to the orchestra and conductor, in a gesture of thanks.

This was not just another good performance of a difficult work by a fine singer, conductor Amos said. It was an historic accomplishment. "This should serve to all of us as a classic example of the power of the mind, and even more significant, our perception that the so-called 'mentally handicapped' people may have hidden abilities as yet untapped by the rest of us," Amos wrote in a weekly column.

Voice teacher Barbara Hasty was thunderstruck by how impeccably Gloria performed. Howard was right. She *could* do it. Barbara felt bad for ever doubting it. Howard's belief in Gloria, his unwavering confidence in her ability, made Barbara realize that people only do as well as they're expected to do. Howard's expectations continued to be high, and Gloria continued to live up to them. This was, Barbara said, the biggest musical accomplishment of Gloria's life.

Gloria knew it.

"Mom and Dad," she said later, "that was the hardest work I've ever done."

With one major life goal accomplished, the Lenhoffs turned their attention to their next, greatest, and perhaps most difficult task: finding a place where Gloria could live the rest of her life without them. A place that would give them peace, knowing she would be well cared for, and happy, after they were gone. They had put off looking for a permanent home for Gloria because she insisted she didn't want to leave them, but Howard was in his seventies now and Sylvia wasn't far behind. They knew they could procrastinate no longer.

Howard had a short but nonnegotiable list of musts. Health and safety must come first. It must be a place where Gloria could continue to grow musically, where she could keep taking voice and accordion lessons, where she could continue to perform publicly. It didn't much matter if it was a small group home or a large institution, if it was a religious establishment or a secular one; it just must be a place that would give Gloria access to the one pure joy of her life: music.

Doug Miller had served with Howard on the Williams Syndrome Foundation board. His daughter, Liz, attended the Belvoir music camp, and was now living at the Baddour Center in Senatobia, Mississippi, a town of just seven thousand people a half hour south of Memphis. Baddour was a Christian "residential ministry" for 180 adults with mild to moderate mental retardation. While the Deep South's Bible Belt wasn't exactly where Howard and Sylvia had envisioned Gloria living out her life, Baddour gave them a glimmer of hope: It had a traveling choir called the Miracles that was on the road thirty weekends a year. Gloria could become a member of the choir, learn a whole new repertoire, and perform all over the country. The Millers sent the Lenhoffs a video about Baddour featuring the Miracles singing; Gloria saw it and surprised her parents by saying, "That is where I want to live."

The Lenhoffs visited in the spring. Baddour sprawled across 120 acres garlanded with lakes and flower gardens, and they were charmed by the lushness of the Mississippi countryside. A red brick chapel—with whitewashed doors and great stained-glass windows of Jesus and his disciples—was the heart of Baddour life, a place for Bible study and worship that always erupted in song. Fanning out from the chapel were fourteen ranch-style group homes for people like Gloria who needed constant supervision, and four duplex apartment buildings for those who could live more independently. As the Lenhoffs poked around, a familiar-looking face peeked out from a window: a woman with Williams syndrome, smiling at them. There was a stout administrative building with a fitness center, a community life building with a movie theater, a kitchen big enough for cooking classes. There was a medical clinic and a greenhouse complex where many residents worked raising flowers. If it was dedicated only to music and had a place for parents to live, it would have been very close to the ideal vision that Howard had held in his mind for years.

The Miracles choir existed, Baddour said, to glorify and give honor to our Lord, Jesus Christ; to spread the Word of God throughout the country; to demonstrate the potential of adults with mental retardation; and to tell the story of the Baddour Center. The Lenhoffs attended a rehearsal and were impressed by choir director Chris Antill, a religious, humorous man who joked with the singers who obviously loved him. The pianist was a very talented resident, David Trivitt, who flawlessly accompanied Gloria on "The Holy City" without a single rehearsal. The choir director called for the Baddour senior staff to come and watch; there was no doubt that Gloria was a Miracle. This is it, Gloria told them. This is the place.

Howard and Sylvia's hearts would have been lighter if they could have found a comparable Jewish center, but one did not exist. They congratulated Gloria on her new home, and set out to make Mississippi their new home as well.

The Lenhoffs, now retired from UCI, went back to California to wrap up their old lives and to prepare for the move. They soon got an excited call from choir director Chris Antill: the Miracles had been asked to perform in a showcase of specially abled musicians at the Kennedy Center in Washington, DC, but only if they could be booked with a related half-hour program. Why not Gloria? Gloria could do a wonderful thirty minutes on stage at the Kennedy Center, he said.

The Lenhoffs happily accepted, flew to Baltimore, and drove to Washington to meet up with the Miracles. There was little time for rehearsal. Dressed in professional black and white, Gloria joined the Miracles on the Millennium Stage in the Grand Foyer. Gloria promptly launched into "The Lord's Prayer," accompanied only by the elegant piano work of Baddour resident David Trivett. Choir members joined hands and bowed heads. Then they all launched into the upbeat "We Are His Miracles," "Sing the Lord a Joyful Song," and other songs of praise, before stepping up to the microphone and introducing themselves, one by one, to the crowd. "Thanks everyone for being here," Gloria said to applause.

Then she reemerged as soloist, ready to show her chops. She launched into the song that so moved the crowd at the Berkshire Hills fund-raiser: "Somewhere." Opera was next, with "Deh vieni, non tardar," Susanna's aria from *The Marriage of Figaro*, taunting Figaro for doubting her fidelity; then the Hebrew folk song "Let There Be Peace"; and an intense version of "The Impossible Dream" that took on added meaning as she hit the high note on "To reach the unreachable star." She squinted hard into the spotlight's glare as the audience exploded in applause. She bowed, rose, bowed, rose again. "Reach the unreachable star, everyone!" she said as the applause failed to subside. "God bless. Thank you."

The Lenhoffs sold their home in Costa Mesa and bought a condo in nearby Oxford, Mississippi, not far from Baddour and Gloria. Before they left California, they arranged a grand farewell at Congregation B'nai Israel; people came from as far away as San Diego and Thousand Oaks to hear Gloria sing her musical good-bye. One was her bus driver when she was in grammar school. Another couple was at her bat mitzvah. Gloria chanted part of the Friday evening religious services before about 125 of them, then harmonized with a choir. She thanked them for their love through the years, for believing in her, and for listening to her music. People started to cry, and that choked Gloria up as well.

I will see you again, she assured them. You are all my friends. I love you and I will be back.

On September 11, 2001, Howard and Sylvia set off for Mississippi in a packed car, with heavy hearts. News stations faded in and out as they drove, delivering the latest on the tragedy in New York and Washington, DC. Howard couldn't help but think that their lives were changing in many, many ways that day.

Gloria had moved into a group home at the Baddour Center. It was a difficult adjustment, learning to share a room with a roommate for the first time, doing her share of household chores, eating unfamiliar foods like collard greens and grits. Gloria was homesick. Howard and Sylvia had been her shadows throughout her entire life; rarely were they more than a few steps away. Now she was on her own. They gave her a cell phone that dialed only two numbers: theirs and 911.

It was time to let go. Howard and Sylvia were satisfied knowing Gloria had a place to call home. They were in their seventies, and finally had an empty nest. Through Gloria's gift, and their unwavering insistence, opportunities were truly opening up for the disabled. They believed that Gloria, by perfecting her skills and performing widely, helped stimulate the growing interest in music among Williams families, an interest that offered hope and meaning to their lives. The next generation of Williams people would have more choices than Gloria had had, and their futures would be brighter. Not a bad accomplishment for a girl who was never supposed to amount to much.

It was a warm, sunny day in June 2003 when the Berkshire Hills Music Academy held its first graduation. More than two hundred people gathered on its gently rolling lawn to see John, Tori, Chris, and the others don green caps and gowns, march in to "Pomp and Circumstance" (played on bagpipes), then stride across the stage to accept their certificates in a thunder of whoops and howls. Sharon Libera cried. It was beyond a dream come true to see John in cap and gown, enjoying the genuine graduation experience that she never thought he'd have. Bob Ackley learned how to laugh and cry at the same time as Tori leapt into the air, hooting and howling, as she accepted her certificate. The Lenhoffs watched it all, greatly pleased.

Aerosmith's Brad Whitford gave the commencement address. It was just a few years ago that he had met Gloria at Kay Bernon's house and went on to play "Sweet Emotion" and "I

Don't Want to Miss a Thing" with Williams musicians at the Berkshire Hills fund-raiser. Now, a practice room bore his name, and his wife's name, and what once seemed like a distant vision had heft and form and texture. Nowhere did the words "Dream on, dream until your dreams come true" seem to fit so perfectly as at Berkshire Hills on that day.

An emotional Sharon Libera took the podium. "As we gather here in this beautiful setting in the Connecticut River valley, with its spectacular westward view toward the river, with the Holyoke Range rising above it, it is good to remember that this section of the river is known as the Pioneer Valley. When it was first explored by the English colonists, there was no overland route, no road, from Boston. It was a task for the boldest among them who would leave the safe coastline and come up the uncharted river, the pioneers. Today it is my privilege, at this first graduation of the first class from this pioneering institution, to introduce the pioneers whose imagination and devotion led us to this moment. It is appropriate that we celebrate the vision of those extraordinary friends whose work paved the way for the Berkshire Hills Music Academy."

A visionary award went to Nancy Goldberg, for having the foresight, faith, and determination to start a music camp for Williams people, when so few believed they had any musical potential.

Another went to Sally Reis, the professor of educational psychology at the University of Connecticut, who was inspired by Chris Lawson to help develop the music-centered teaching methods used at Berkshire Hills.

But foremost among these visionaries, Sharon said, was the Lenhoff family.

"Sylvia and Howard Lenhoff went beyond meeting the ordinary challenges of raising a child with a disability, to recognize and nurture the artistic education of a profoundly gifted person, their daughter, Gloria," Sharon said. "They fought to gain opportunities for her that were equal to her talent. And, once they learned, when she was thirty-three years old, that her disability was a syndrome shared by many, they fought just as hard for all those other families whose children deserved a musical education. . . . Howard envisioned an academy of musical arts for people with intellectual disabilities. It was a pioneering idea, a school that would allow those who were differently abled to develop their gifts for their own fulfillment as well as for the good of society, and many of us would not be here today were it not for his very great powers of persuasion. It is he who inspired Kay Bernon with the passion to take up the challenge of creating this new kind of school.

"Gloria, for her part, has exemplified the life of a serious artist. She has taken voice and instrument lessons for many years, always improving, always taking on new and dazzling challenges. She has performed widely, sharing a special joy with her audiences, small and large. She has donated the proceeds of her concerts to the Williams Syndrome Foundation, which has supported several scholarships that have helped students to attend this academy. She has been an example to many, showing that a person with intellectual disabilities can make a great contribution to others."

Sharon raised a simple trophy and smiled. "To the Lenhoff family, for originating, developing, and promoting the academy concept. For spearheading the work of the Williams Syndrome Foundation. For cofounding the Williams Syndrome Music and Arts Camp. For countless articles, interviews, concerts, and media appearances. For your tireless advocacy and inspiring example, we present this Visionary Award on behalf of the grateful members of the Berkshire Hills Music Academy."

Howard felt a swell of emotion in his throat as applause crackled and he made his way to the podium. He waited for the noise to die down. "A Jewish tradition is to refer to our parents as teachers," he finally said. "In various Hebrew prayers, we refer to 'my father, my teacher' or to 'my mother, my teacher.'

Today, however, we want to acknowledge 'our daughter, Gloria, our teacher.'

"Gloria has taught us what true love is. To be compassionate to others who are less fortunate than ourselves. But most of all, she has taught us to recognize that everyone has something different to offer society. . . . Gloria taught us, as your children taught you. Thank you, Gloria."

{*coda*}

Meghan Finn's father has done a lot of thinking about what this all means. "There's no question that we, as parents, have influence on our children," Kevin Finn said. "But there's an awful lot of that raw material — I don't want to say 'programmed,' but *established* at birth. When I see Meghan, what strikes me is how much we don't understand."

The haunting conclusion scientists are reaching from their studies of Williams people is that chemistry, indeed, is destiny. Things as complex as personality, behavior, and thought processes are deeply rooted in genetics. Not just for Williams people. But for all of us. Barbara Pober, a clinical geneticist at Yale University School of Medicine, said she wouldn't be surprised if something as specific as a preference for chocolate ice cream is somehow coded in our DNA. Her non-Williams patients do not hug her and tell her they love her; but, almost without fail, her Williams patients do. Scientists now believe Williams is much more prevalent than previously thought, occurring in one of every 7,500 births, rather than one of every 20,000.

Williams is a scientific mystery that offers a window into the mechanics of the human mind. Salk researcher Ursula Bellugi said it is one of the most interesting things she has ever come across. The fact that a tiny number of specific genes are missing gives scientists an unparalleled opportunity to directly link genes to brain and behavior. It's an extremely tricky area—as controversial claims of the discovery of the "thinking gene" showed—but many believe it is the future, and the frontier, of science. Which genes dictate the architecture of the brain? How do they do it? How is that enigmatic organ wired, and how does it rewire itself to deal with deficits? People with Williams syndrome will help answer these questions, and the next decade of research will enhance our understanding of the human condition by light-years, many researchers believe.

We'd love to be able to say that science finally understands exactly how Williams syndrome occurs, and exactly how the brain systems that process music and language and facial information are preserved when so much else is severely damaged. We'd love to be able to say that scientists now know exactly which genes are responsible for the outgoing personality and spatial intelligence deficits and empathy that are so characteristic of Williams people. But we can't. Science just isn't there yet. And among scientists, disagreement still runs hot on exactly what role genes and environment play in Williams syndrome, especially regarding language and music abilities. Some researchers feel there has been too much exaggeration and not enough serious research.

But the huge disparity between strengths and weaknesses in Williams people leads to one inescapable conclusion: Intelligence isn't a monolith. It's much more fluid than scientists have long believed, and there's a great deal of "functional independence" in the brain's underlying systems. You can be good at language and lousy at reasoning. You can be good at music and unable to multiply numbers. It all boils down to this, UCI researcher Greg Hickok said: "We don't have a unified mind. It's composed of different computational systems. We're built up out of a bunch of pieces. To understand the mind, we need to understand not only those components, but how they interact to give rise to the illusion of a single, unified, whole."

Howard believes that Williams people prove our whole definition of intelligence is wrong. "I don't call them 'retarded,'" he said. "I call them 'mentally asymmetric.' Williams people have a real musical intelligence, often surpassing that of normal individuals. Many other mentally handicapped populations might have untapped potentials waiting to be discovered—if only researchers, and society, would take the time and trouble to look for and cultivate them."

The lesson that Gloria, Meghan, Alec, John, Brian, Tori, Chris, and other Williams musicians teach is that mentally handicapped people can not only do spectacular things, but also that they can do some even better than "normal" people.

The music camp idea pioneered by Howard and Sharon has caught on. They've been held in Detroit, San Antonio, Nashville, and Connecticut. The University of Texas, San Antonio, has started one, as well as the University of Connecticut and Vanderbilt University. The Berkshire Hills Music Academy hosts a music camp, and music camps are now in Ireland, Japan, and Spain as well. Many of the Belvoir Terrace and Berkshire Hills graduates are now working, at least part-time, with music.

"It's like music is their language—the sound of music is their way of thinking and feeling," said Meghan's father. Or, as Dr. Jonas Salk so bluntly said after hearing Gloria sing at a Christmas concert, "I've always believed that talent was a birth defect."

♪　♪　♪

Gloria has settled into her new, semi-independent life in Mississippi. Singers in the Deep South are duty-bound to honor traditional spirituals and the blues; Gloria takes lessons from masters of these genres and is having a ball discovering new types of music. She has an accordion teacher and a voice teacher, and continues work on her repertoire and technical skills.

Such songs can sound quite eclectic, sung by an operatic soprano and played on the accordion.

Gloria sang Christian hymns with the Miracles for a time, and now works for Baddour's development office. She is on constant call to sing at Baddour events, and to entertain visitors at the Baddour Center; she takes computer classes, exercises regularly, helps her home coordinator with cooking and other domestic chores, and attends several major conferences each year to sing, while Howard serves as a keynote speaker.

In Mississippi, Howard and Sylvia felt compelled to do something about the poverty they saw all around them. They began the Guardian Angel Initiative through an efficient local charity called Youth Opportunities Unlimited. It has raised some $5,000—including proceeds from Gloria's performances—and aims to help at least five hundred impoverished children by providing the bare essentials needed to attend public school: clothes, shoes, school supplies, and educational field trips. The children live in one of the poorest areas of Mississippi—the Delta counties of Coahoma, Quitman, Tallahatchie, and Panola.

In the twilight of Howard's life, top cognitive and genetic scientists have accepted him as a peer, and they wrote chapters for the scholarly book on Williams he edited along with Colleen Morris and Paul Wang: *Williams-Beuren Syndrome: Research, Evaluation and Treatment.* It was published by Johns Hopkins University Press in 2006, and was inspired, as always, by Gloria.

On the side, Gloria studies classical music at the University of Mississippi and cantorial singing at a synagogue in nearby Memphis. As chance would have it, the synagogue is right across the street from the Opera Memphis offices. Howard had traded e-mails with the opera's artistic director, Michael Ching, hoping it could work with Gloria on a fund-raiser for Baddour. After a cantorial lesson, Howard and Gloria marched across the street and asked to see Ching. Ching was in his office and invited them in. Gloria sang some Puccini arias, Ching was impressed, and said he'd see what he could do about working somehow with Gloria.

In fall 2005, Opera Memphis would be staging *Samson et Dalila*, an Old Testament story recounting how Hebrew strongman Samson is seduced by conniving Philistine Dalila. Samson confesses the secret of his strength, Dalila betrays him, and they all are destroyed. A large and versatile chorus is the backbone of the opera, which is sung in French; the chorus portrays long-suffering Hebrews in one act, and Philistines drunk with victory in another. Ching thought about what people might have been like thousands of years ago, and concluded they were probably very much like people today. It's very likely that there were people like Gloria in those communities. He had a bold idea: why not take a chance and cast her Gloria in the chorus?

Singing in a concert is one thing. Functioning in a stage show is something else completely. Gloria had never done any stage acting. She never had to enter and exit many times on cue, or follow complicated stage directions. She had never been treated as a full professional in a full professional company. Could she do it? Howard, excited but nervous and raising the bar ever higher, insisted she could.

Ching did two things to accommodate Gloria that he didn't usually do. First he made an extensive rehearsal CD for her, so she could learn the music. While he was at it, he made CDs for the rest of the cast as well, and it proved to be a breakthrough: It helped them learn the music as much as it helped Gloria. Ching decided rehearsal CDs would become a regular feature. Then Ching assigned a mentor to accompany Gloria on stage and off: experienced soprano Sharon Dobbins. Sharon had been teaching music to kids with learning difficulties for years, but never had she met anyone like Gloria.

Sharon had always taken pride in how quickly she learned music, but it stunned her that Gloria was even faster. At the first rehearsal Gloria attended, half the cast clutched note cards and sheet music, but Gloria knew everything by heart. "This is going to blow your mind," Sharon said, "but I felt I was with a colleague. She knows her music so well. She was more prepared than many of them on stage."

Rehearsals began in August 2005 for performances in October and November. Howard and Sylvia again put everything in their lives aside, rented an apartment in Memphis so Gloria could attend daily rehearsals, and lived there for more than a month.

From a costuming perspective, there were problems. The wardrobe department had trouble finding robes small enough to fit Gloria: she was half the size of some of the other singers. And no one who lived during biblical times wore eyeglasses, and certainly not eyeglasses as thick as Gloria's. Howard and Sylvia considered getting Gloria contact lenses, but that would have been a logistical nightmare for her. Instead, Gloria got new, frameless glasses that were nearly invisible from the audience.

During the performance, those who watched very closely might have seen Sharon whispering instructions to Gloria: "Smile, smile, smile," to stop Gloria's gaze from settling into a fixed stare. "Raise your arms. . . . Turn your hands out. . . . Climb the stairs. . . . Let's run off stage."

Gloria's balance and sense of depth perception were sorely lacking, so Sharon learned to always be the one closest to the edge of the stage or the stairs; if one of them was going to fall, it was not going to be Gloria.

Sharon put a chair backstage so Gloria could rest between entrances, but during one rehearsal, Sharon turned around and Gloria was gone. Sharon panicked. She ran out of the wings and found Gloria wandering the halls; in all the excitement, Gloria needed to use the restroom. They missed an entrance, but Sharon learned a lesson: before and after each and every appearance on stage, they visited the facilities and made themselves comfortable.

Cast members tried to include Gloria in their conversations;

she made a game of reading their palms and telling them how long their life lines were. Gloria adored the music, the camaraderie, the costumes, the hot lights, the applause. Artistic director Ching was a bit worried that she might stand out, but she blended into the chorus wonderfully and added real power to the soprano section, he said. He invited her back for a spring production marking Opera Memphis's fiftieth anniversary, and she was scheduled to sing in the chorus of *Il Trovatore* in 2007.

It was a groundbreaking thing for Opera Memphis to do. If other professional music companies would be as bold as Ching's, a new world of possibilities could open up for Williams people. There is hope that this may happen: a small opera company in northern Mississippi, Como Opera, has invited Gloria to sing in its chorus for future productions as well.

But a crisis of sorts looms for the Berkshire Hills Music Academy. It was relicensed by the Massachusetts Department of Mental Retardation as a "work/community support program" and a "residential support program" in 2004, gaining a two-year certification with distinction. But the reality for its graduates, as Gloria well knows, is that it's still very difficult for Williams syndrome people to find work in the field of music. As a stop-gap measure, Berkshire Hills has started a new one-year program for its graduates called Music in Careers; it lets them return for a third year for more intensive training in performance or musical education and therapy. It postpones, for one more year, the inevitable crash into the brick wall of opportunity. Despite all their training and hard work, it's still very difficult for talented Williams people to go find work in music once school is over.

Tori Ackley's father, Bob, is trying in his own way to remedy that. He's working on an idea for a "Troupe House," to be built on the Berkshire Hills campus, which would be a permanent home for some performers. They'd live together, make music together, raise awareness together, grow older together, much as Howard had always envisioned. The troupe would perform at nursing homes, daycare centers, senior centers, church events, corporate functions, public schools, city functions, fund-raisers, wherever its full-time staff could book it. The third-year students at Berkshire Hills would work with the troupe as well, maybe join it someday. Without more opportunities like Gloria had at Opera Memphis, Bob just can't see any other way for Williams students to turn their music into career paths. "You can't be in school forever," Bob Ackley said. "Tori is twenty-three. If this doesn't happen, Tori will come home and it will be over."

Howard would love to see a village surrounding Berkshire Hills, something much like Baddour. It could help people with disabilities in all aspects of their lives while focusing on music. There would even be places nearby where parents could live, because, like the Lenhoffs, many wouldn't want to be far from their children. But all of that is still a vision. Despite all of Howard and Sylvia and Gloria's hard work, despite all of Sharon and Kay and Nancy's hard work, despite all the flash and sizzle that Williams syndrome has generated among scientists and the media, this is still true: Williams people are far more ready for the world than the world is ready for them.

{an open letter from
Howard Lenhoff}

"*This may seem strange to you, but in some ways I feel it was for the best that Becky died before I did. At least I know that she had the loving care of her mother throughout her life.*"

Haunting words. They were told to me when I was offering condolences to a mother who had just lost her fifty-six-year-old daughter. Fate answered her greatest fear, one that plagues virtually all parents of handicapped children: *After we die, will our child be able to live in good health in a safe and happy place and still be able to grow as an individual?*

That concern takes a special twist for parents of children born with Williams syndrome, who have a love and talent for music. Will music continue to be a major part of the lives of our children, and will they continue to develop as musicians with opportunities to share their love and their music with audiences?

Teri Sforza does a great service as she brings the reader into the world of the beautiful and talented Williams people and their parents, highlighting the success of the music camp, the establishment of the Berkshire Hills Music Academy, and the advances by researchers in our understanding of the syndrome. What a stunning beginning for dealing with a condition that was first

261

reported only in 1961, and which did not attract international attention until the early 1990s.

My views on what the next years could add to the story of Williams syndrome stem from a number of facets of my background: I am a father of a Williams syndrome music savant, a scientist who has investigated absolute pitch in Williams musicians, and a social activist. From those diverse perspectives, I have come to believe that the Williams story provokes significant questions in three areas and offers some tantalizing clues and possible models for the future. Further, I am convinced that following those clues will yield rewards extending well beyond the disabled community.

First, as a father, I empathize with the frustrations of other parents: "We want to be with our kids as long as we can; we want them to be near family." Most tell me that they might be able to scrape up enough loans and money to give them two years at the Berkshire Hills Music Academy, but they could not come up with $30,000 yearly for the rest of their child's adult life, the amount charged by most private residential institutions for the intellectually disabled.

There is no single solution. I suggest one model in which the Berkshire Hills Music Academy could provide the core for a unique residential community of houses or condominiums located near the academy. It would offer two types of residential arrangements. One would be homes for retired or semiretired parents and their Williams children. The other would be dormitories or smaller group homes for the Williams adults after their parents are no longer with them. Those would be run according to state regulations. Most residents would be able to pay for their care through combinations of Social Security, Supplemental Social Security Income (SSI), and family resources. Regardless of whether they lived on the premises with their parents or in a dormitory or group home, the Williams people would have most of their daily social and music activities centered *at* the music academy.

Next, as a scientist, how would I advise an agency that funds music research on Williams syndrome? The focus needs to be on investigating the spectacular accomplishments of Williams people, rather than on what they cannot do. For example, that some Williams people have ceiling levels of absolute pitch, can recall in seconds long and complex melodies and lyrics—some in many foreign languages—is a phenomenal ability. Various parts of the brain function at a high level to allow Williams people to perform in this manner. Whereas any one of the twenty missing genes may interrupt many cognitive processes in Williams people, large numbers of genes and interconnected nerve cells are doing something right. To brush aside those surprising abilities and call them "compensatory" responses in efforts to "make up" for their disabilities is unscientific.

I urge that scientists examine anecdotal observations of enhanced musical traits observed in Williams people, such as rhythm, timbre, and recall in order to rigorously define and quantify those abilities. Without numbers, scientists will not be able to unlock the secrets that an understanding of Williams musicality might reveal about the brain, and particularly about the "critical periods" during which the brain allows each of those musical traits to develop. Examination of the timing of the critical periods in musical individuals having other syndromes may yield further insights. Like much basic research with atypical participants, the results garnered may give us a new understanding of how the normal brain operates.

In those investigations, the rationale for what constitutes a proper set of control participants may need to be reevaluated. For example, are we on the right track in comparing measurements of Williams people to those obtained from either normal or other cognitively disabled populations, such as those with Down syndrome, who are either the same chronological age or who have the same IQ? Some current studies suggest that Williams adults may retain many of the incredible learning attributes characteristic of normal children in their first six years of life. Perhaps those normal children should be the control participants in studies of the musical abilities of Williams people.

A final useful area of research might approach questions of the musical abilities of Williams people as they age. Will they follow the same trends of aging as do regular populations, or will they differ? For example, do the vocal chords of Williams people deteriorate at the same rate as they do in normal people? At what ages do Williams people lose their amazing capacities to retain and recall melodies? What might this tell us about aging and learning in the general population?

Finally, my role as an activist in getting music on the Williams syndrome agenda that Teri Sforza skillfully describes has been only part of the battle. In that journey we parents encountered an unexpected sinister aspect of human nature—a nearly universal bias against the retarded. One need only watch television, go to the movie theater, or listen to popular comedians to hear the constant stream of clichéd "retard" jokes. Some are cruel, such as that by a popular major network TV talk-show host comparing retarded people to dogs. Jokes at the expense of the retarded seem to have no limits; they are even bandied about by individuals who themselves are objects of bias—for instance, members of the African American and gay communities. I tire of hearing "senior citizens" at their retirement declare with a laugh, "Now I am retarded."

Unfortunately, it is not only the everyday uninformed person who unthinkingly finds such barbs witty. Well-respected research scholars have written: "It appears that absolute pitch is typical of either musical precociousness or mental retardation. So if you have it, be sure it is for the right reason." Equally troubling is a peculiar blind spot of some researchers in the field of music cognition who dismiss research demonstrating that people with Williams syndrome have high levels of musical abilities. If people having a low IQ possess those abilities, does it seem somehow to those investigators to diminish the importance of their own research in establishing music as one of the highest forms of cognition?

How can you, the reader, assist Williams people in using their musical gifts to combat the widespread negative attitudes toward them and retarded individuals in general? As your starting point, recall that when Gloria, or Alec Sweazy, or Tori Ackley, or other skilled Williams syndrome musicians have the opportunity to perform for audiences, those gifted individuals are able to change by 180 degrees the misconceptions regarding the abilities of those labeled retarded by society.

The problem is finding opportunities for them to perform. Sylvia and I learned early that it is not easy to find mainstream venues for performances by our Williams musicians. We even have the services of an excellent agent. Once potential clients find out Gloria is intellectually disabled, however, she is often passed over. Program planners, we've found, sometimes feel their audiences will be uncomfortable with cognitively disabled artists and believe audiences would rather be entertained by a physically disabled comedian making fun of her or his own disability.

Readers may learn of possible opportunities for Williams performers that arise in your community and your religious, civic, and professional organizations. When you do, try contacting the Berkshire Hills Music Academy, the Williams Syndrome Foundation, and the Williams Syndrome Association (see appendix A). Ask for the name, phone number, and address of Williams syndrome musicians who live nearby and are able to perform varied programs for those audiences.

Our positive experiences at scholarly and professional meetings, and with such pioneering groups as Opera Memphis, the Tifereth Israel Community Orchestra (San Diego's community orchestra), and the San Diego Master Chorale, have taught us a great deal about what Maestro Michael Ching describes as the benefits of "Mutual Mainstreaming." He was surprised and gratified that as Gloria was integrated into the Opera Memphis chorus, both she and the ensemble learned and gained from each other. We need to find and call upon more such superb leaders in the worlds of the arts, entertainment, and science to provide arenas for Williams musicians to perform, to delight, and to influence hearts and minds. It is a win-win situation. We all stand to reap the rewards.

A HOW-TO FOR PARENTS OF MUSICAL WILLIAMS SYNDROME CHILDREN

by Howard and Sylvia Lenhoff

- **How do we get started?** Williams syndrome children at a very early age show signs of enjoying music. Though they may be able to focus on most tasks for but a few minutes, they may listen to music for extended periods of time. By the time they are four to five years old, some may have developed a repertoire of pieces that they recognize or sing. These may be simple children's songs, but some may be complex classical works. From talking with many Williams parents, we understand that this ability to appreciate and perform music appears at an early age, but its development depends heavily upon parental help.

- **What should we do?** Three things: First, let your child experience a wide variety of music. Ever since our daughter Gloria was an infant she has been exposed to music. Sometimes we simply played loud classical pieces because we could not tolerate her constant screams caused by colic pains. When she was a toddler, she had a number of musical toys, including such simple instruments as a small wooden xylophone. As she grew older, she had her own radio, tape recorder, and supply of cassettes. Later we noticed that when Gloria was alone in her room watching TV, she would often search for channels that either had music or foreign-language programs. All these experiences, we believe, contributed to her love of music and her musical skills.

- **What next?** Once your child shows an interest in music, encourage him to sing and perform for and with family and friends. Some of the happiest moments of Gloria's childhood for all of us, once she overcame her colic and started to sleep at night, were the many times she and her younger brother performed for the family after supper. At first the cleared kitchen table became our stage as they would take turns singing. Later we, an amateur guitarist (HL) and pianist (SL), would try to accompany them. As they got older, Gloria became proficient at the accordion and we became superfluous. To this day she has retained virtually all these songs of her childhood, whereas we eventually have forgotten most of them.

- **Do we need to purchase any musical instruments?** Nothing major at first, but you should get a variety of simple rhythm instruments. For example, when Gloria performs at home for family and friends, we help motivate her and also get everyone involved by passing out simple rhythm instruments that we have collected over the years. Here are some of the things we do: shake a toy or professional tambourine; beat two wooden sticks; click toy castanets; shake maracas or a variety of rattles; ring clusters of bells; beat on a gourd or on a toy drum; shake Hawaiian bamboo sticks; rub blocks of wood with sandpaper stapled to them; and, as a last resort, strike pots and pans with wooden spoons! At a minimum, rhythmic clapping by all provides an incentive to our budding performers. Because we raised Gloria before the modern computer age, we are not familiar with many of the new simple electronic instruments available. Karaoke tapes are also useful to teach your child new songs and to sing with accompaniments. We have been using this technique for several years.

- **Selecting an instrument.** Find one that the child enjoys and that fits her physical, motor, and cognitive limitations. Voice training may be the best way to start, but many children excel in classical piano, electronic keyboard, guitar, violin, saxophone, clarinet, organ, and others have uncanny ability on the drums.

- **Selecting a teacher.** Do not get someone who is rigid. Do not insist at the beginning required reading of musical notation. Try a bright and warm high school student or college student. Advertise in school newspapers. Later, try and get a more professional teacher who also is flexible. Remind the teacher of teaching one step at a time, and of some of the cognitive and motor problems that Williams musicians face. They do better in one-on-one situations with the teacher, rather than in group classes. Most of their learning takes place through hearing and imitating.

- **Using technology.** The most successful music lessons for Williams people are recorded on tape or digitally, with the student practicing daily while listening to the recorded lesson. For more complex music, like songs in a variety of unfamiliar foreign languages, some special recording techniques work extremely well. For example, to teach a folk song in a foreign language, record a native speaker singing the song, then enunciate slowly a two- or three-word phrase of the song and sing it, until the song is completely recorded. Insert a few silent periods on the tape to allow time for the student to repeat those phrases. By listening to such tapes and practicing daily, some Williams students can learn songs in a foreign language rapidly and retain those songs in their repertoire virtually indefinitely.

- **How old should they be to start?** It doesn't matter if they're six, sixteen, or thirty-six—all those ages are perfect because the window of opportunity to learn music is jammed in Williams syndrome and remains open into adulthood.

- **Role of parents.** Parents need to be supportive, providing encouragement and praise. Those Williams syndrome musicians who excel usually have highly committed parents. There is a lot of prejudice out there. Parents need to advocate for their child, even in school and church and synagogue choirs. And they need to help their child succeed in these circumstances. Parents are also the ones who often arrange performances for the child. But they also have to learn how to stand back and let the child have his own life.

{*Appendix B*}
RESOURCES

Williams Syndrome Association
   P.O. Box 297
   Clawson, MI 48017-0297
   Phone: (800) 806-1871 and (248) 244-2229
   Web site: http://www.williams-syndrome.org

Williams Syndrome Foundation
   University of California
   Irvine, CA 92697-2300
   Phone: (949) 824-7259
   Web site: http://www.wsf.org

Berkshire Hills Music Academy
   48 Woodbridge Street
   South Hadley, MA 01075
   Phone: (413) 540-9720
   Web site: http://www.berkshirehills.org

{*bibliography*}

PRELUDE

Bishop, Jane. Translation of arias from Mozart's *Le Nozze di Figaro*. http://www.aria-database.com/cgibin/ariafinder.pl?222 (accessed January 2002).

Holoman, D. Kern. Plot for Mozart's *Le Nozze di Figaro*. http://hector.ucdavis.edu/Music10/RecList/MozArias/MozMFar.htm (accessed January 2002).

Sforza, Teri. "Music from the Soul: A Puzzling Mental Handicap Suggests Personality, Behavior Are Rooted in Genes." *Orange County Register*, August 9, 1998.

CHAPTER 1

Crawford, Kit. "Whatever Happened to Dr. Williams?" http://www.wsf.org/family/news/whatever.htm (accessed January 2002).

Howard Hughes Medical Institute. "An Introduction to HHMI." http://www.hhmi.org/about (accessed January 2002).

Mallery, Richard, et al. "Blaise Pascal." http://oregonstate.edu/instruct/phl302/philosophers/pascal.html (accessed December 2001).

Williams, J. C. P., B. G. Barratt-Boyes, and J. B. Lowe. "Supravalvular Aortic Stenosis." *Circulation* 24 (1961): 1311–18.

CHAPTER 2

Bartleby.com, Great Books Online. "Song of Songs. The Holy Bible: King James Version." http://www.bartleby.com/108/22/ (accessed March 2005).

Jewish Women's Archive. "JWA-Jewish Women in Your Life-Bat Mitzvah Guide." http://www.jwa.org/discover/inyourlife/batmitzvah /index.html (accessed January 5, 2006).

Melitz, Leo. "The Opera Goer's Complete Guide: The Magic Flute." http://www.brainyencyclopedia.com/encyclopedia/t/th/the_magic_ flute.html (accessed April 2005).

Menszer, John. "Two Yiddish Songs." Audio file, http://www.holocaust survivors.org/cgi-bin/data.show.pl?di=record&da=recordings &ke=9 (accessed March 2005).

Pearson Education. "Favorite Opera Stories." http://www.infoplease .com/ipea/A0153765.html (accessed April 2005).

CHAPTER 3

Alda, Arlene, and James Maas. *Bravo, Gloria!* Produced by Psychology Film Unit, Cornell University. PBS documentary, broadcast May 1, 1988.

Christian, Susan. "Perfect Pitch: Gloria Lenhoff Is a 'Musical Savant' Who Sings and Plays Beautifully but Can't Understand Mathematics." *Los Angeles Times*, December 23, 1990.

Fisher, Marla Jo. "Still Growing at 40." *Orange County Register*, October 4, 2005.

Huff, Steve. Translation of Strauss's "Morgen!" http://www.planethuff .com/steve/archives/000238.html (accessed January 2006).

Lenhoff, Howard. "Activist Shifts Focus to Nurture Jewish Retarded." *Orange County Jewish Heritage*, January 28, 1994.

———. *From Conception to Birth.* Dubuque, IA: Kendall/Hunt, 1993.

Luna, Claire. "Their Graduation Comes with Fear: Disabled Adults Leave Special Programs for a World of Uncertainty." *Los Angeles Times*, June 23, 2002.

Taylor, Steven J. "Disabled Workers Deserve Real Choices, Real Jobs." http://www.accessiblesociety.org/topics/economics-employment/shelteredwksps.html (accessed May 2005).

CHAPTER 4

Alda, Arlene. "About Arlene Alda." http://www.arlenealda.com/bio.htm (accessed February 2005).

Alda, Arlene, and James Maas. *Bravo, Gloria*. Produced by Psychology Film Unit, Cornell University. PBS documentary, broadcast May 1, 1988.

Basheda, Lori. "All the Right Notes: The Hi Hopes Celebrate 30 Years of Making a Place for Themselves in the World." *Orange County Register*, May 26, 2002.

Gordon, Jean. "The Gift of Music: Woman with Williams Syndrome Sings Perfectly in 30 Languages." *(Jackson, MS) Clarion-Ledger*, March 13, 2004.

Hinch, Robin. "Daring School Gives Retarded Kids Hi Hopes." *Chicago Tribune*, February 22, 1985.

Hoffman. Jan. "Hi Hopes: 'Impossible' Not in Dictionaries at University for Gifted Retarded." *Los Angeles Times*, April 23, 1988.

Kopetman, Roxana. "Handicapped but Gifted Adults Get Anaheim Fine Arts Campus." *Los Angeles Times*, March 16, 1986.

———. "Retarded Adults Prove Value of Their Talents: Anaheim Council OKs Site for Hope University, but Some in Neighborhood Protest Vehemently." *Los Angeles Times*, March 3, 1986.

Maas, James. "Interests." Cornell University Department of Psychology. http://comp9.psych.cornell.edu/people/Faculty/jbm1.html (accessed February 2005).

Pierson, Robin. "Instruments of Hope: Paul Kuehn." *Orange County Register*, May 24, 1987.

———. "A Mind for Music: Mentally Retarded Members of Hi Hopes Share a Special Talent, the Mysterious Ability to Tap Their Brains for Chord Changes and Song Lyrics." *Orange County Register*, May 25, 1987.

Reingold, Edwin M. "They All Have High Hopes: A Unique School Develops the Gifts of the Mentally Impaired." *Time*, March 2, 1987.

Takahama, Valeria. "Mentally Retarded OC Woman's Talents Get Big 'Bravo!' in Documentary." *Orange County Register*, April 28, 1988.

Williams Syndrome Association. "What Is Williams Syndrome?" http://www.williams-syndrome.org/forparents/whatiswilliams.html (accessed April, 2005).

Wong, Herman. "Hi Hopes Are Soaring with Success: Talented Handicapped Grab Public Attention." *Los Angeles Times*, April 18, 1987.

———. "Retarded Woman's Life, Musical Gifts Inspire Public TV Special." *Los Angeles Times*, April 29, 1988.

CHAPTER 5

Bellugi, Ursula. "Biography." Salk Institute for Biological Studies. http://www.salk.edu/faculty/faculty/details.php?id=3 (accessed January 2006).

Bellugi, Ursula, et al. "Dissociation between Language and Cognitive Functions in Williams Syndrome." In *Language Development in Exceptional Circumstances*. London: Churchill Livingstone, 1988.

Bellugi, Ursula, H. Sabo, and J. Vaid, "Spatial Deficits in Children with Williams Syndrome." In *Spatial Cognition: Brain Bases and Development*. Hillsdale, NJ: Lawrence Erlbaum Associates, 1988.

Bellugi, Ursula, Paul P. Wang, and Terry L. Jernigan. "Williams Syndrome: An Unusual Neuropsychological Profile." In *Atypical Cognitive Deficits in Developmental Disorders: Implications for Brain Function*. Hillsdale, NJ: Lawrence Erlbaum Associates, 1994.

Beuren, J., J. Apitz, and D. Harmjantz. "Supravalvular Aortic Stenosis in Association with Mental Retardation and Certain Facial Appearance." *Circulation* 26 (1962): 1235–40.

Blakeslee, Sandra. "Odd Disorder of Brain May Offer New Clues." *New York Times*, August 2, 1994.

Broman, S., and J. Grafman. *Atypical Cognitive Deficits in Developmental Disorders: Implications for Brain Function*. Hillsdale, NJ: Lawrence Erlbaum Associates, 1994.

Christian, Susan. "Song of a Savant: Gloria Lenhoff's Musical Talents Overshadow Her Other Limitations." *Los Angeles Times*, December 27, 1990.

Finn, Robert. "Different Minds." *Discover*, June 1991.

Jernigan, T. L., and Ursula Bellugi. "Anomalous Brain Morphology on Magnetic Resonance Images in Williams Syndrome and Down Syndrome." *Archives of Neurology* 47 (May 1990): 529–33.

———. "Neuroanatomical Distinctions between Williams and Down Syndromes." In *Atypical Cognitive Deficits in Developmental Disorders: Implications for Brain Function*. Hillsdale, NJ: Lawrence Erlbaum Associates, 1994.

Lenhoff, Howard, et al. "Williams Syndrome and the Brain." *Scientific American*, December 1997.

Mervis, Carolyn B. "Williams Syndrome: 15 Years of Psychological Research." *Developmental Neuropsychology* 23 (2003): 1–12.

Schultz, Robert, David Grelotti, and Barbara Pober. "Genetics of Childhood Disorders: Williams Syndrome and Brain-Behavior Relationships." *Journal of the American Academy of Child and Adolescent Psychiatry* 40, no. 5 (May 1, 2001): 606–609.

Sforza, Teri. "Brain Variances Found in Williams Persons." *Orange County Register*, August 9, 1998.

von Arnim, G., and P. Engel. "Mental Retardation Related to Hypercalcaemia." *Developmental Medicine and Child Neurology* 6 (1964): 366–77.

Williams, J. C. P., B. G. Barratt-Boyes, and J. B. Lowe. "Supravalvular Aortic Stenosis." *Circulation* 24 (1961): 1311–18.

CHAPTER 6

Dickey, Tom. "A Rare Drummer with Rare Challenges." *Presbyterian Record*, November 2002.

Doeff, Gail. "Dairy Foods Top 50." *Dairy Foods*, July 1994.

Donovan, William J. "Texas Firm to Acquire Garelick Farms: Suiza Foods Corp., a Dallas-Based Company, Will Pay about $400 Million for the Dairy, Water and Bottle Companies Garelick Farms Owns." *Providence (RI) Journal-Bulletin*, June 24, 1997.

Finn, Robert. "Different Minds." *Discover*, June 1991.

Jacobus, Georgianne. "Message from the Late Georgianne Jacobus." http://www.wsf.org/medical/literature/layreader/jacobus.htm (accessed January 2005).

Morris, C. A., et al. "Adults with Williams Syndrome." *American Journal of Medical Genetics Supplement* 6 (1990): 100–101.

Morris, C. A., et al. "Natural History of Williams Syndrome: Physical Characteristics." *Journal of Pediatrics* 113 (August 1988): 2.

Morris, Colleen. University of Nevada School of Medicine Genetics Program. http://www.unr.edu/med/dept/Genetics/Research.html (accessed January 2005).

Ordonez, Franco. "Charity Is Flourishing on Bernon Family Tree." *Boston Globe*, May 13, 2004.

Patton, Natalie. "Reaching for the Stars." *Las Vegas Review-Journal*, November 22, 1998.

Robinson, John. "Berendt's Book Adds a Little Sex to Noble Syllabus." *Boston Globe*, October 11, 1994.

Stoke-on-Trent Tourist Information Center. "Welcome to Stoke-on-Trent." http://www.visitstoke.co.uk (accessed April 2005).

Swartz, Brian. "Grant's Dairy Builds First New Dairy Seen on East Coast in 20 Years." *Bangor (ME) Daily News*, September 16, 1995.

CHAPTER 7

American Museum of Natural History. "Jesup North Pacific Expedition." http://www.amnh.org/exhibitions/Jesup/fieldletters/ (accessed May 2005).

Belvoir Terrace. "History of Belvoir Terrace." http://www.belvoirterrace.com/int_history.shtml (accessed March 2005).

"Case History of a Child with Williams Syndrome." *Pediatrics* 75 (1985): 962–68.

Klein, A. J., et al. "Hyperacusis and Otitis Media in Individuals with Williams Syndrome." *Journal of Speech and Hearing Disorders* 55 (May 1990): 2.

Lenhoff, Howard. "Real-World Source for the 'Little People': The

Relationship of Fairies to Individuals with Williams Syndrome." *Nursery Realms: Children in the Worlds of Science Fiction, Fantasy and Horror*. Athens: University of Georgia Press, 1999.

Libera, Sharon. *For the Love of Music*. Williams Syndrome Foundation. Documentary videotape, 1992.

Reis, Sally, et al. "Williams Syndrome: A Study of Unique Musical Talents in Persons with Disabilities." *National Research Center on the Gifted and Talented Newsletter*, Fall 2000. http://www.gifted.uconn.edu/nrcgt/newsletter/fall00/fall002.html (accessed October 2005).

Suzuki Association of the Americas. "Every Child Can Learn." http://www.suzukiassociation.org/parents/twinkler/ (accessed April 2005).

Suzuki Music Academy. "The Basic Principles of the Suzuki Method." http://www.suzukimusicacademy.com/Suzuki-methodLinksIndex.html (accessed April 2005).

Tinnitus FAQ. "Hyperacusis." http://www.bixby.org/faq/tinnitus/related.html#causes (accessed January, 2006).

von Arnim, G., and P. Engel. "Mental Retardation Related to Hypercalcaemia." *Developmental Medicine and Child Neurology* 6 (1964): 366–77.

Williams College. "Morris K. Jesup." http://www.williams.edu/library/archives/buildinghistories/jesup/benefactor.html (accessed May 2005).

CHAPTER 8

Adams, Noah. "A Combination of Mental Retardation and Mental Gifts." *All Things Considered*, National Public Radio, December 19, 1994.

Boucher, Geoff. "Beautiful Mystery: They Struggle to Tie Their Shoes and Make Change, but They Can Master Music and Languages. It's All Part of the Williams Syndrome Riddle." *Los Angeles Times*, August 26, 1994.

Center for the Study of Complex Systems. "Neuropsychology." http://cscs.umich.edu/~crshalizi/notebooks/neuropsychology.html (accessed February 2005).

Curran, M. E., et al. "The Elastin Gene Is Disrupted by a Translocation Associated with Supravalvular Aortic Stenosis." *Cell* 73 (April 9, 1993): 159–68.

Don, Audrey J., Glenn E. Schellenberg, and Byron P. Rourke. "Music and Language Skills of Children with Williams Syndrome." *Child Neuropsychology* 5 (1999): 3.

Ewart, A. K., et al. "Hemizygosity at the Elastin Locus in a Developmental Disorder, Williams Syndrome." *Nature Genetics* 5 (1993): 11–16.

Ewart, A. K., et al. "A Human Vascular Disease, Supravalvular Aortic Stenosis, Maps to Chromosome 7." *Proceedings of the National Academy of Sciences* 90 (1993): 3226–30.

Lenhoff, Howard. "The Nature of Elastin." http://www.wsf.org/medical/literature/layreader/elastin.htm (accessed November 2001).

Morris, C. A., et al. "Supravalvular Aortic Stenosis Cosegregates with a Familiam 6;7 Translocation Which Disrupts the Elastin Gene." *American Journal of Medical Genetics* 46 (1993): 737–44.

Rorden, Chris. "Neglecting Half of the World." http://www.sph.sc.edu/comd/rorden/neglect.html (accessed February 2005).

Toppman, Lawrence. "Detweiler Calls on Life Lessons: Writer's Spiritual Experiences Influence Characters." *Charlotte (NC) Observer*, September 29, 2001.

CHAPTER 9

Mattoon, Donna B. "A Disability Marked by Musicality." *Berkshire (MA) Eagle*, August 29, 1994.

Toppman, Lawrence. "He Was Born to Make Music — and Make It His Own." *Charlotte (NC) Observer*, August 3, 1997.

Warshaw, Dalit. "Williams Syndrome: Pondering the Complexities of a Musical Gift." *Juilliard Journal*, November 1996. http://www.wsf.org/music/musiced/muponder.htm (accessed November 2001).

CHAPTER 10

Angier, Natalie. "A Gallery of Human Oddities That Are, After All, Human." *New York Times*, August 23, 1998.

Bellugi, Ursula, Gregory Hickok, and Wendy Jones. Letter to the editor. *Science*, October 13, 1995.

Evans, Julian. "Journey to the Centre of the Psyche: Dr. Oliver Sacks's Travels in the Human Mind Make Compelling Reading." *Guardian* (UK), October 18, 1996.

Karmiloff-Smith, Annette, et al. "Exploring the Williams Syndrome Face-Processing Debate: The Importance of Building Developmental Trajectories." *Journal of Child Psychology and Psychiatry* 45 (2004): 7.

Karmiloff-Smith, Annette, et al. "Is There a Social Module? Language, Face Processing and Theory-of-Mind in Individuals with Williams Syndrome." *Journal of Cognitive Neuroscience* 7 (Spring 1995): 2.

Mervis, Carolyn B. "Williams Syndrome: 15 Years of Psychological Research." *Developmental Neuropsychology* 23: 2003.

Rosetta Pictures. *Mind Traveller*. http://www.rosetta.co.uk/mind .htm (accessed April 2005).

Rowe, M. L., A. M. Becerra, and Carolyn B. Mervis. "The Development of Empathy in Williams Syndrome." Presented at the Biennial Conference of the Society for Research in Child Development, Tampa, FL, April, 2003.

Sacks, Oliver. "Don't Be Shy, Mr. Sacks: William's Syndrome." BBC documentary film, *Mind Traveller* series, produced by Rosetta Pictures, 1996.

———. Letter to the editor. *Science*, May 5, 1995.

Sullivan, K., E. Winner, and Helen Tager-Flusberg. "Can Adolescents with Williams Syndrome Tell the Difference Between Lies and Jokes?" *Developmental Neuropsychology* 23 (2003): 1, 2.

Tager-Flusberg, Helen. "Social Cognition in Williams Syndrome." National Science Foundation conference on Separability of Cognitive Functions: What Can Be Learned from Williams Syndrome? University of Massachusetts, Amherst, August 23, 2001.

Tager-Flusberg, Helen, Jenea Boshart, and Simon Baron-Cohen. "Reading the Windows to the Soul: Evidence of Domain-Specific Sparing in Williams Syndrome." *Journal of Cognitive Neuroscience* 10 (September 1998): 5.

Tager-Flusberg, Helen, and Kate Sullivan. "A Componential View of Theory of Mind: Evidence from Williams Syndrome." *Cognition* 76 (2000): 59–90.

Thomas, Melissa L., Angela M. Becerra, and Carolyn B. Mervis. "Empathy in Four-year-old Children with Williams Syndrome." National Science Foundation conference on Separability of Cognitive Functions: What Can Be Learned from Williams Syndrome? University of Massachusetts, Amherst, August 23, 2001.

Toppman, Lawrence. "Detweiler Calls on Life Lessons: Writer's Spiritual Experiences Influence Characters." *Charlotte(NC) Observer*, September 29, 2001.

CHAPTER 11

Blakeslee, Sandra. "Researchers Track Down a Gene That May Govern Spatial Abilities." *New York Times*, July 23, 1996.

CBS News, *60 Minutes* Program Facts, http://www.cbsnews.com/stories/1998/07/08/60minutes/main13503.shtml (accessed February 2005).

Dare, Eric. "Unusual Trio of Piano, Clarinet and Soprano." *West Briton* (UK), December 11, 2003.

Detweiler, Craig. *A Highly Musical Species.* Documentary film, produced by EO Productions, 1996.

Frangiskakis, J. M., et al. "LIM kinase-1 Hemizygosity Implicated in Impaired Visuospatial Constructive Cognition." *Cell* 86 (July 12, 1996): 1.

Goetinck, Sue. "Gene May Be Tied to a Specific Mental Capacity." *Dallas Morning News*, July 15, 1996.

Hickok, Gregory. "Research Interest in Learning and Memory." http://www.cnlm.uci.edu/hickok.htm (accessed October 2005).

Lenhoff, Howard. "Preservation of a Normally Transient Critical Period in a Cognitively Impaired Population: Window of Opportunity for Acquiring Absolute Pitch in Williams Syndrome." In *Toward a Theory of Neuroplasticity*. Philadelphia: Taylor and Francis, 2000.

Lenhoff, Howard, et al. "Williams Syndrome and the Brain." *Scientific American*, December 1997.

Lenhoff, Howard, Olegario Perales, and Gregory Hickok. "Absolute Pitch in Williams Syndrome." *Music Perception* 18 (Summer 2001): 4.

Massachusetts Institute of Technology. "Program Notes for 'Shepherd on the Rock.'" http://web.mit.edu/king-lab/www/people/silverwood/ 10-02_Program_notes.html (accessed November 2005).

McNatt, Glenn. "Bach's 'Easy' Pieces Teach a Hard Lesson about Music, Not Piano Playing." *Baltimore Sun*, January 14, 1996.

Osborne, Lucy, and Barbara Pober. "Genetics of Childhood Disorders: XXVII. Genes and Cognition in Williams Syndrome." *Journal of the American Academy of Child and Adolescent Psychiatry* 6 (June 1, 2001): 40.

Palca, Joe. "Scientists Identify Specific Cognitive Gene." *All Things Considered*, National Public Radio, July 11, 1996.

Patton, Natalie. "Reaching for the Stars." *Las Vegas Review-Journal*, November 22, 1998.

Sacks, Oliver. "Don't Be Shy, Mr. Sacks: William's Syndrome." BBC documentary film, *Mind Traveller* series, produced by Rosetta Pictures, 1996.

Safer, Morley. "A Very Special Brain: Scientists Believe by Studying People with Williams Syndrome, They May Be Able to Solve Some of the Mysteries of the Brain." *60 Minutes*, CBS News, broadcast July 5, 1998.

Scheiber, Dave. "Music Lights a Fire." *St. Petersburg (FL) Times*, September 6, 1998.

Schmidt, Dan. "Perfect Pitch." http://www.dfan.org/pitch.html (accessed March 2005).

Warshaw, Dalit. "Williams Syndrome: Pondering the Complexities of a Musical Gift." *Juilliard Journal*, November 1996, http://www.wsf .org/music/musiced/muponder.htm (accessed November 2001).

CHAPTER 12

Levitin, Daniel. "Biography." http://ego.psych.mcgill.ca/levitin.html/ bio.html (accessed October 2005).

Levitin, Daniel, and Ursula Bellugi. "Musical Abilities in Individuals with Williams Syndrome." *Music Perception* 15 (1998): 4.

Safer, Morley. "A Very Special Brain: Scientists Believe by Studying People with Williams Syndrome, They May Be Able to Solve Some of the Mysteries of the Brain." *60 Minutes*, CBS News, broadcast October 19, 1997.

CHAPTER 13

Berkshire Hills Music Academy. "Our Mission." http://www.berkshirehills
.org/about.htm (accessed March 2005).

Bohemian Opera. "Translations of *La Bohème* Arias." http://www
.bohemianopera.com/aria1.htm (accessed January 2006).

Hatfield, Julie. "Party Lines: A Filling Tribute to Peace in Ireland at
Boston Marriott." *Boston Globe*, November 20, 2000.

Kahn, Joseph P. "Learning in Concert at a New School for People with
Disabilities, Music and Life-Skills Classes Work in Harmony."
Boston Globe, December 3, 2002.

Kramer, Suki. "Finer Than Silk." *Holyoke (MA)*, September 9, 1999.

Reis, Sally, et al. "Music and Minds: Using a Talent Development
Approach for Young Adults with Williams Syndrome." *Exceptional
Children* 3 (March 22, 2003): 69.

Reis, Sally, et al. "Williams Syndrome: A Study of Unique Musical Talents in Persons with Disabilities." *National Research Center on the
Gifted and Talented Newsletter*, Fall 2000. http://www.gifted.uconn
.edu/nrcgt/newsletter/fall00/fall002.html (accessed October 2005).

Williams Syndrome Foundation. "Residential Academy." http://www
.wsf.org/music/berkshire.htm (accessed April 2005).

Wistariahurst Museum. "Good Silk Is Always Good Property: A
Skinner Silk Exhibit." http://www.wistariahurst.org/silk.htm
(accessed January 2006).

CHAPTER 14

BBC online. "Sergey Rachmaninov." http://www.bbc.co.uk/music/profiles/
rachmaninov.shtml (accessed January 2006).

Brunner, Liz. "New School Uses Music to Teach Life Skills." Segment
for the Boston Channel News, WCBV Channel 5, broadcast January 29, 2002.

Kahn, Joseph P. "Learning in Concert at a New School for People with
Disabilities, Music and Life-Skills Classes Work in Harmony."
Boston Globe, December 3, 2002.

Kramer, Suki. "Finer Than Silk." *Holyoke (MA)*, September 9, 1999.

Lenhoff, Howard. "Preservation of a Normally Transient Critical Period in a Cognitively Impaired Population: Window of Opportunity for Acquiring Absolute Pitch in Williams Syndrome." In *Toward a Theory of Neuroplasticity*. Philadelphia: Taylor and Francis, 2000.

Lenhoff, Howard, Olegario Perales, and Gregory Hickok. "Absolute Pitch in Williams Syndrome." *Music Perception* 18 (Summer 2001): 4.

Levitin, Daniel, and Ursula Bellugi. "Recent Research on Williams Syndrome and Music." National Science Foundation conference on Separability of Cognitive Functions: What Can Be Learned from Williams Syndrome? University of Massachusetts, Amherst, August 23, 2001.

Teachout, Terry. "What Was the Matter with Rachmaninoff?" *American Jewish Committee Commentary*, June 1, 2002.

Wikipedia. "Prelude in C-sharp Minor (Rachmaninoff)." http://en .wikipedia.org/wiki/Prelude_in_C-sharp_minor_(Rachmaninoff) (accessed January 2006).

Chapter 15

Amos, David. "Music Notes." *San Diego Jewish Times*, June 1999, http://www.wsf.org/family/news/1999.htm (accessed January, 2006).

———. "Music Notes." *San Diego Jewish Times*, August 4, 2000.

Baddour Center. "History." http://www.baddour.org/about/history.cfm (accessed November 2005).

Kennedy Center. "Millennium Stage." http://www.kennedy-center .org/programs/millennium/pafe.html (accessed January 2006).

Kuenning, Geoff. "Barber: Knoxville, Summer of 1915." http://www .lasr.cs.ucla.edu/geoff/prognotes/barber/knoxville.html (accessed November 2005).

Ledbetter, Steven. "Samuel Barber." Pro Arte Chamber Orchestra of Boston, http://www.proarte.org/notes/barber.htm (accessed November 2005).

Lieberman, David Isadore. "Notes on Knoxville: Summer of 1915." http://www.loudounsymphony.org/notes/barber-knoxville (accessed November 2005).

Royko, Kevin. "South Hadley Music School Has First Graduation." *Daily Hampshire (MA) Gazette*, June 4, 2003.

Sforza, Teri. "Friends Are Sorry to Lose Joyful Voice of Gloria Lenhoff." *Orange County Register*, January 16, 2001.

———. "A Song Fill's Gloria's Soul." *Orange County Register*, January 7, 2001.

St. Madeleine Sophie's Center. "History." http://www.stmsc.org/pages/history.html (accessed December 2005).

Wilkens, John. "With a Song in Her Heart." *San Diego Union-Tribune*, June 24, 1999. http://www.wsf.org/family/news/sdtrib.htm (accessed January 2006).

CODA

Farrell, John. "A Worthy 'Samson and Delilah.'" *Press-Telegram* (Long Beach, CA), February 24, 2005. http://u.presstelegram.com (accessed December 2005).

Lisle, Andria. "Delightful Gloria: Soprano with Williams Syndrome One of Stars at Opera Memphis." *Memphis Business Journal*, October 28, 2005. http://www.wsf.org/family/news/delightfulgloria.htm (accessed January 2006).

Morris, Colleen. "Williams Syndrome." http://www.geneclinics.org/profiles/williams/details.html (accessed January 2006).

Schultze, Lucy. "Local Singing Star to Be Featured in Opera Memphis." *Oxford (MS) Eagle*, October 21, 2005. http://www.wsf.org/family/news/schultze_operamemphis.htm (accessed January 2006).

Sforza, Teri. "Music from the Soul: A Puzzling Mental Handicap Suggests Personality, Behavior Are Rooted in Genes." *Orange County Register*, August 9, 1998.

{index}